I0790455

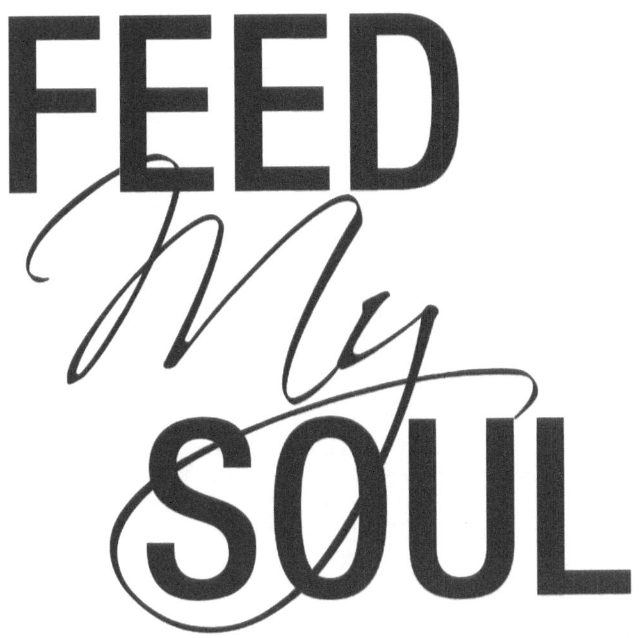

Finding *True Peace with* Food, Movement, Rest, *and* Body Image

KRISTEN BUNGER, MS, RD

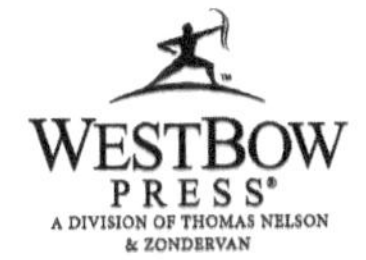

WESTBOW
PRESS®
A DIVISION OF THOMAS NELSON
& ZONDERVAN

WestBow Press books may be ordered through booksellers or by contacting:

WestBow Press
A Division of Thomas Nelson & Zondervan
1663 Liberty Drive
Bloomington, IN 47403
www.westbowpress.com
844-714-3454

ISBN: 978-1-6642-8141-7 (sc)
ISBN: 978-1-6642-8142-4 (hc)
ISBN: 978-1-6642-8143-1 (e)

Library of Congress Control Number: 2022919276

Print information available on the last page.

WestBow Press rev. date: 01/06/2023

CONTENTS

Dedication

To every person who has struggled to make peace
with food and their body. May this book bless you
on your journey to freedom and may you see the
goodness of God in the land of the living.

INTRODUCTION

Every time I meet a new client, I ask for the details of their story. I want to know where their issues with food began and how they have manifested. Each story resonates with me. Each and every one of us has struggled with eating, movement (exercise), rest, and body image in some way, and we all have *really good reasons for the struggle.*

Eating disorders, disordered eating, "yo-yo" dieting, body image dissatisfaction, and the like are merely unhealthy and irrational ways of meeting healthy and rational needs. Whatever your reason for picking up this book, it is a good reason. More than likely, in some way, you have been using food and your body to meet healthy, rational, normal, shared-by-all-of-humanity, God-given needs. Behavior change is much less intimidating if we look at those behaviors in the light of normalcy and grace. It might feel like you have been filled with shame and unrest for so long, and you are finally ready for a change.

Before I discuss behavior change in more detail, I will define some of the struggles I mentioned above.

Important Definitions

Disordered eating - Eating in a way that is disorganized, chaotic, or irregular. It is inconsistent, and it does not honor the body's needs. The reason for disordered eating might be due to a lack of time, energy, money, or boundaries. It causes stress, worry, angst, and overall discomfort (both emotionally and physically).

"Yo-yo" dieting - Frequently switching from one diet to another. Adhering to food restrictions, food rules, or dieting trends in an effort to control your body. It is characterized by dramatic changes in behaviors around food and drastic up-and-down weight changes. It results in weight gain and shame when the diet inevitably "fails." "Yo-yo" dieting causes physical and mental damage, and distrust of the body.

Body image dissatisfaction - The feeling that your body needs to change in some way in order for you to feel adequate. It is relying on your body to partially or fully satisfy needs that it is unable to and not designed to satisfy. Body image dissatisfaction often causes so much distress and unhappiness that the person is pushed to extreme dieting, eating disorders, or plastic surgery to change their body.

Eating disorders are best defined in the *Diagnostic and Statistical Manual of Mental Disorders, Fifth Edition* (2022). They are typically diagnosed in a psychiatric setting. If you are suffering from an eating disorder, this book should be used as one of many resources to help with eating disorder recovery. Treatment for an eating disorder should involve a full team, including a physician, therapist, dietitian, and psychiatric provider who specialize in the treatment of eating disorders.

Some of you may say, "I don't think my behaviors are *that* drastic," or " There is no possible way I can think about food and my body in a peaceful way." If this is the case, I pray you will give me the chance to impart a fresh perspective to you. My goal is for you to finish this book being able to see yourself the way God sees you.

Topics That Will be Discussed

First, I'm going to show you how things can be different. There are four main areas in which I would love for you to attain more peace as we journey together:

1. *Peace with food*- Being able to eat in a consistent and peaceful way. Seeing food as nourishment and enjoyment rather than a way to cope with emotional needs.
2. *Peace with movement*- Moving for enjoyment rather than out of obligation. Giving yourself grace when movement doesn't happen.
3. *Peace with rest* - Allowing your body time to be renewed when needed without feeling guilty.
4. *Peace with your body* - Seeing your body as God's wonderful creation and not assigning value to yourself based on how your body looks.

As a clinical dietician, I have had the privilege of leading many people to peace in these areas. In the chapters that follow, I will teach you practical, simple ways to think about these areas differently.

I have been practicing nutrition for fifteen years, but I have also been a follower of Jesus most of my life. My love for God and my conviction that Jesus is the Way, the Truth, and the Life impact everything I do, including my work. Therefore, I am going to include many scriptures and biblical truths that have helped me and my clients in these areas over the years.

At the end of the day, my belief is that we are made in the image of God for His glory. When we don't know that (or forget it), we will naturally try to gain fulfillment elsewhere. All the other "fillers" just leave us wanting more. I want to help you find peace with food, movement, rest, and your body. But I also want to remind you that no person, no diet, no fitness level, and no accomplishment in life will ever fulfill you like Jesus can.

Coming to Terms With Your Fear

Almost all of my new patients experience a mixture of emotions when starting this journey with me. Moving things around in your life to make room for lasting changes can make you feel happy, sad, excited, and hesitant all at the same time. If you are feeling nervous, know it is totally expected, and you are in good company.

The potential for failure is scary. I recently had a client say to me, "I know I am doing well right now, but it never lasts. I always fall off the wagon with this stuff." I gently reminded her of her dieting history and her account of "trying every diet" before starting nutrition therapy with a registered dietitian. I asked her to consider that this time might be different because the approach is so different. She was now actively trying to heal her relationship with food and be kind to herself rather than engaging in restrictive and militant patterns to change her body. I immediately felt the fear drain from her body as she began to feel hope again.

You might relate to my client above, who so humbly said, "This is great, but I am scared. I don't want to fail again." You may have lots of experience with the dieting cycle. It starts successfully for a time with whatever diet you are trying, then you have a setback, gain weight again, try again, have more setbacks, and eventually give up. It's common to see a rebound in weight gain after the diet is over. This is always the result of restriction and rigidity.

Here, in these pages, you are going to read what my clients hear when sitting in my office. I offer safe, empathetic, science-based, grace-based, and presence-of-God-filled advice. We will explore how grace-driven effort can lead to the changes in your life that you have been seeking.

I will warn you, though. Diets are flashy, glamorous, and sexy to some extent. They are fast and promise big results in record time. This journey in which I will guide you is not flashy, and it doesn't happen overnight.

The process of getting back to balance and health could be compared to a long-lasting covenant marriage. One of my clients, who had been married for fifteen years to a man she loved deeply, admitted to me one day, "our marriage is good, but it takes a lot of work." When she was surprised that "doing simple, little things every day to take care of my body feels very hard sometimes," I asked her to think of her marriage and the commitment she had made to her spouse. I reminded her of the depth, goodness, security, and intimacy she had nurtured with him all those years. She got my point and said, "So this romance with my body is going to take work, but it's going to be forever and awesome. Is that what you are telling me?"

"Exactly, my friend."

Support from Loved Ones

This book by itself is not enough to bring order into your relationship with food, movement, rest, and body image. I pray it will be a helpful tool, but you may need more. Only you can determine if and what "more" you will need, but here are a few suggestions.

As a trusted ally to my clients, I have heard many stories and observed many people's lives. I have watched the progression from disordered eating to successful recovery over and over again. One of my biggest observations over the years is this: the clients who have strong support systems always do better than those who don't. It is not just sometimes, it is *always*.

You might be married or in a committed relationship. You might be living with your parents or other family members. You may have very close housemates. Or, you might live alone but have dear friendships. Whatever your current situation, it is time to sit down with your loved ones and let them know that you are on a journey to better self-care and health. This might seem unnecessary or silly, but the boundaries that you will inevitably need to set are going to affect your loved ones. It would be a courtesy to let them in on the changes they can expect to see in you.

Additionally, you will need a safe person with whom you can share your struggles and who can provide accountability.

This book contains much more than "drink more water and eat

more fiber." We are going to talk about motivation, heart matters, family wounds, and true healing. If I succeed, you will laugh, cry, and be forever changed by these pages. And someone else besides you needs to witness it. This process is too important and too good to keep to yourself. So, take a moment to say a prayer and think about who may be a safe person to talk to about this matter. Make a plan to talk to them soon; reach out, send a text, and invite them in. Tell them the ways they can support you and allow that to evolve as you go.

Professional Support

While it's my opinion that seeking support from loved ones is necessary, professional support may or may not be something you will need. Before you skip over this section because you think reading this book is the same thing as professional support, let me just say, it's not the same. There is a big difference between reading a book written by a professional and sitting in the presence of a professional week after week while their whole focus in that hour is on you and no one but you.

I cannot speak highly enough about nutrition therapy and psychological counseling. I know some might say that I am biased, but my bias does not come from a selfish place. Unfortunately, I won't ever meet most of you. But I have worked with hundreds of clients in my career, and I have seen miracles occur in their lives. I am not saying you are only going to get what you want out of this process if you hire a dietitian and a therapist, but I am saying that you may need that level of support.

This book is intended to be a truth-filled resource to come back to over and over. It will help you to remember the basics and to understand the simplicity of what is needed for success in this area. But many of you may want or need more support. If that is the case, please get it. You are never going to look back on this season and say, "I really wish I hadn't gotten more education and emotional support for myself." It will likely be very much the opposite.

What Kind of Support Do You Need?

So how do you know if you need more support than this book and a few trusted family members and/or friends? Well, let me ask you, do you feel like you need more support? If you know in your gut that you do, now is the time to get it. If you don't know, the knowledge may come as this process unfolds. Here are some signs that you would benefit from the professional support of a dietitian and therapist:

1. You are following the advice given in this book but need more accountability to be consistent and successful.
2. You are getting a lot out of this book as you read, but you would like a professional to help you process the information and provide further education.
3. If you feel overwhelmed, highly triggered, or re-traumatized by anything in these pages, stop reading and seek further help.

There is a list of resources at the back of the book that can help you decide which direction to go and where to look for help. No matter how much support you need during this process, I pray you will realize you are worthy of receiving the help and make it happen for yourself.

Changing Thought Patterns

Each of us have foundational and philosophical thoughts about food, movement, rest, and body image that have been formed in us from infancy. But the beautiful thing about growing up and becoming mature in all things is that we get to decide what thoughts we keep and what thoughts we "throw out." Your philosophies about food, movement, rest, and body image might be in need of an overhaul. In each chapter, you will be challenged to replace your disordered thoughts with biblical and philosophical truths.

I encourage you to grab a pen and underline what you like on each page. Add a question mark on what you are not sure about, and write fears or criticisms next to the parts that you feel like rejecting. Be *honest without judgment* toward yourself as you work through these concepts and these areas of your soul that are hopefully ready for change. As you dive into each page, be open to hearing your soul's fears and try to identify where those fears are coming from.

Body and Soul

During the first few years of my career as a dietitian, I worked at an inpatient eating disorder treatment facility. One particular client wrote me a letter at the end of her stay with us. She wrote, "Kristen, you fed my body, but you also fed my soul." It was the highest compliment I had ever received. That day, I heard God's call to write this book. Twelve years later, here we are.

The biggest idea God has shown me over the course of my career is that you can have everything "right" as far as eating and exercise, but it doesn't mean anything without God in your life. You can have all the knowledge, wisdom, and teaching this world has to offer, but those things will never fill the God-shaped hole in your heart. God is the giver of life, the Creator, and the One and only One who is able to meet all of our needs. Without Him, we will always be searching for more and wanting for more. With Him, we find our deepest needs met and true satisfaction achieved.

In these pages, I hope you find what you need in the areas of food, movement, rest, and body image. I also hope you learn that no amount of eating the "right" way, moving the "right" way, or changing your body will ever satisfy you the way Jesus can. If He is truly at the center of your life, everything else will fall into place.

If you are still reading, I hope you keep going. My prayer is that you will wrestle with every word in the following chapters. Test and try each concept and take what you need from these pages. It would be my greatest joy to sit with each of you and ask you what you think, what you love, what you hate, and what you are afraid of. But I will settle for this book because I believe that if you begin this journey toward peace with food and body, you will be forever changed for the better.

PART I

*Disordered Eating, Movement,
Rest, and Body Image*

CHAPTER 1

The Beginning of Disorder

The righteous person may have troubles, but the Lord delivers him from them all.

—Psalm 34:19

Consider the contents of your junk drawer. You know the one. Mine is the drawer in the corner of my kitchen, right next to the fridge. There are chip clips, a box of rubber bands, lip balm, magic tricks, notepads, pens, a teething necklace, coupons, dry-erase markers, a postage stamp, and a few pens. If you look at that list, none of those things are actually useless (except maybe the magic tricks). They all have a job to do. They just need to be put in order so I can find them when I need them and so they can accomplish their purpose.

Some pens do need to go to "pen heaven" because they have been out of ink for two years, and I just don't have the sense to walk over to the garbage can and throw them away after I discover they don't work. Instead, I just shake the pen and try to write with it again, and when it doesn't work, I throw it back in the drawer and try another one. Don't laugh. I know you have done it too. But I digress.

The kitchen junk drawer might be a silly analogy, but it can be likened to our beliefs about food, movement, rest, and body image. The thoughts get jumbled up in the "junk drawer" of our mind, and we don't often take the time to sort through, organize, and throw out what doesn't actually work.

But here's the beautiful thing: this organization might take time and a lot of effort, but the result of order is always peace. Always. It's time to look at the "junk drawer" where all your beliefs about food, movement, rest, and body image lie jumbled, find them a home (or put them in the garbage can), and be at peace.

When did the "Junk Drawer" Become So Disorganized?

The junk drawer in my kitchen wasn't always disorganized, and neither was your relationship with food, movement, rest, and body image. Many times I will hear from clients, "I don't know why I feel this way about my body. I don't know why I eat the way I do and have the fears I have. I don't even know when this started." Every epic story has a beginning, and your story is no different. At some point, you began to receive messages that you, the food you eat, your movement, your body, or all of them, were not okay.

While some clients can't pinpoint a start to their "junk drawer" disorganization, others can tell me the exact moment that their peace in these areas left them. It usually happened before they were ten years old, and for some, it happened before they were five years old. The specific moment might have involved trauma, a hurtful comment, or a neutral comment that was perceived as criticism.

Whether you can remember the specific moment or not, we all come to realizations at some point in our life about our bodies and food. Some of these realizations are neutral and factual, and some of them are dark and judgmental. If you have never explored when disorder began for you, it's time. Ask yourself these questions:

- When did all of this start for me?
- When did I begin feeling uncomfortable in my body?

- When did I start believing I had to live up to unrealistic standards?
- When did I begin to rely on food, and how my body looked to help me cope and control my life?

The purpose of these questions is not to point fingers at anyone or for you to wallow in the pain of the past. The purpose is to start you on the path of healing. Our stories need to be told. Even if you, your therapist, and a few trusted friends are the only ones who witness your full story, it needs to be told. The truth needs to be told because the truth will set you free.

I pray you are beginning to understand more about where your disorder began. If you still feel at a loss with this, or you feel like you only have a few memories to choose from, don't let that get you down. More insight will come as you continue this work. As you become more educated and equipped to do things differently, you will continue to remember moments in your life that have affected you in this area.

Prayer

Lord, help me to remember the significant moments in my story. Help me to know when I began to believe lies about food and my body. Help me pay attention to my thoughts and when I have memories, show me why I am thinking of them. Help me to have courage to be honest about my pain, others who have caused me pain, and areas where I have caused myself pain. Show me, Jesus, where my disorder with food and my body began and give me grace as I begin this journey to health and peace. In Jesus' name, Amen.

Invitation

If you don't have a journal, it would be a great idea to get one. If you would like to, it would greatly enhance your healing process to write about the topics and ideas in each chapter. Additionally, I will ask a lot of questions throughout the book to help you explore what areas of healing are needed. You will likely experience a lot of emotions while reading this book. Journaling can be a very helpful form of releasing difficult emotions. It is also very beneficial to be able to look back and see progress you have made throughout this process. It will help encourage you to keep going!

CHAPTER 2

The Manifestation of Disorder

I consider that our present sufferings are not worth comparing with the glory that will be revealed in us.

—Romans 8:18

An equally important question to "Where did this all begin?" is "How has this disordered thinking manifested in my life?" Another way to say this is, "How was I affected by these negative messages I received early in my life?" It's time to dump out the contents of the junk drawer, start going through it, organizing it, and throwing things away that are not serving us well anymore.

Here is a list of ways disorder could manifest in your life, and a brief definition of what each term means:

- Restriction – Trying to eat as few calories as possible, skipping meals, eating smaller than normal portions, or omitting certain foods or entire food groups.
- Overeating – Eating past the point of fullness.
- Emotional Eating - Eating in response to feeling emotions even in the absence of hunger.

- Bingeing – Eating an extreme amount of food in a short period of time. Often characterized by the feelings of being out of control, disassociated, or "checked out" from the body.
- Calorie counting – Making sure your food intake stays under a certain number of calories each day.
- Purging – Self-induced vomiting after eating. Using other compensatory behaviors or substances to "get rid of" calories like laxatives, diuretics, or over exercising.
- Night eating – Waking up in the middle of the night and eating with or without feeling hunger.
- Mindlessly eating – "Zoning out" while eating and not taking the time to taste or enjoy the food. Often associated with eating in front of a screen.
- Abusing caffeinated beverages – Consuming an extreme amount of caffeine and relying on caffeine for energy instead of food.
- Abusing laxatives – Taking laxative pills for the sole purpose of losing weight, often taking more than the amount indicated on the box.

Listed below are the stories of ten different clients of mine. Take a moment to see if any of their stories resonate with you. These examples might cause you to step back and realize that certain damaging thought patterns were considered normal in the house where you grew up. All names and personal health information have been changed for the privacy of my clients.

Michelle's Story

When Michelle first told me her story, she noted that her disordered eating began with restriction. When she was twelve years old, she lost several close family members in a very short period of time. She described feeling alone, unsure, and emotionally abandoned by her parents. They were grieving so much themselves that they couldn't see her pain too.

She began to restrict food to numb and forget the pain. She also wanted to be invisible and void of emotion. She began to eat very small portions and cut out certain food groups altogether. By the time she was fifteen, her restriction was so severe that she was diagnosed with anorexia nervosa and was admitted to an inpatient treatment facility.

Cynthia's Story

Cynthia came to me after more than twenty-five years of "doing every diet there ever was." She referred to herself as a "chronic dieter" and was coming to me because she just wanted to "learn how to eat and be happy" with herself. She told me, "I am so tired of feeling like I always have to be on a diet." Cynthia started with Weight Watchers when she was fifteen years old. She had joined the program with her mom and had been dieting ever since.

Until working with me, she had never learned how to listen to her body and honor her hunger or fullness cues. She felt like she couldn't eat normally. Most of the time she would restrict her food intake to the point of overeating and bingeing when her hunger was "more than I can bear." She was also fiercely determined to avoid setting her daughters on the same course she had followed. She wanted to model what it looked like to have a healthy relationship with food, movement, rest, and her body.

Isaac's Story

Isaac became my client during his senior year of high school after almost a year of calorie counting and restriction. He had lost seventy-five pounds the prior year. He was beginning to see his performance in school and at work suffer due to a lack of concentration. He was also more irritable, and fearful of adding necessary foods and calories back to his diet. He had begun to believe that he would never be able to be at peace with food again.

Isaac wanted to "not obsess about food all day long and constantly think about what I am going to eat next." At the same time, he had been flattered by many people in his life telling him how great he looked now that he had lost weight. His need for approval and confidence had been so readily met by his eating disorder. It was very hard for him to see the negatives that were outweighing the positives. He had difficulty trusting that he could eat normally and maintain a healthy weight without obsessively controlling his calories.

Jackie's Story

Jackie was in her late twenties when she started seeing me, and she described herself as someone who "has always been big and never really liked healthy foods." After getting to know her better, she began to let me in on her eating schedule, which involved not eating or drinking anything besides coffee until 1:00 or 2:00 p.m. each day. She would eat a small snack or lunch midday, then starting around 5:00 p.m. she would eat the majority of her calories, including a large snack late at night. She described herself as feeling uncomfortably full when going to bed each night and was plagued with terrible sleep due to acid reflux, for which she was medicated.

Jackie never thought of her behaviors as bingeing, but once she was educated on the term, she realized that she had been bingeing and overeating since she was a teenager. She stated she was not hungry in the mornings, and most of the time even felt nauseous when waking up. She was also unsure if she could ever eat "like thin people eat." Jackie admitted she had a great amount of fear and anxiety about the process of healing her relationship with food. She came to see that her judgment of herself and others in regard to food and body image was deeply rooted in trauma, not in truth.

Renee's Story

Renee had just found out she was pregnant with her second child when we began working together. Right away, she owned overeating as a very prominent part of her life. In her teens and early twenties, she had restricted and binged from time to time. When she made meals for her son, she would often not eat with him due to busyness. Then she would become very hungry and overeat snacks before and after dinner. She felt drawn to eat a lot of food during her son's naptime and bedtime because those were her "only moments of peace" during the day.

Renee was very concerned about her unbalanced relationship with food while being pregnant. She was scared that excessive weight gain would complicate her pregnancy and her health. She wanted to take better care of herself and pass down healthy food habits to her children.

Mannie's Story

Mannie's eating disorder stemmed from the trauma he had suffered in childhood. He had already been in intensive outpatient treatment for drug abuse before working with me. He stated he was currently bingeing and purging several times a week. For him, this cycle felt like an "inevitable force I feel I have to do when I feel overwhelmed by my emotions or when I think about trauma from the past."

Mannie didn't feel like he could go to his parents for support when he was upset. He felt like a failure all the time. He wanted to stop his unhealthy eating behaviors, fearing that he would suffer major health issues if he was unable to stop. However, he felt powerless to change.

Jacob's Story

Jacob had been dieting his whole life when he started seeing me in his late forties. A few years prior, he had lost over one hundred pounds following the ketogenic diet. Now, he was terrified to gain it back and therefore was restricting himself heavily during the day. He would wake up in the middle of the night and engage in night eating to satisfy his hunger. He was exhausted from counting, measuring, worrying, and fighting his body. After living in a large body most of his life, he was scared to eat normally, but he was ready for a change.

Hannah's Story

Hannah came to me with a tremendous amount of shame over her eating habits and how those habits had changed her body over the years. She stated that she used food to cope with many uncomfortable situations in life and referred to herself as a "scarfer." She would eat so fast that she wouldn't even taste or experience her food. Often this would lead to overeating or bingeing, but even on her best days she confessed to mindless eating. She no longer found pleasure or satisfaction in food and wanted so badly to slow down and be present with food and her body again.

Rebecca's Story

Rebecca had suffered from chronic restriction since she was in her teens, but by the time she came to see me in her mid-twenties, her eating disorder had severely progressed. She was barely eating anything, drinking less than one water bottle a day, and abusing caffeinated beverages in order to have energy without eating caloric and nutrient-rich foods. Her cycle of food restriction and high volumes of caffeinated beverages caused her to only sleep three to four hours per night. She was ready to start taking better care of her body and feeling better, but she was nervous to "let go" of her unhealthy behaviors.

Veronica's Story

Veronica started working with me after admitting to her spouse that she had been abusing laxatives for more than ten years. She knew it was horrible for her body and was terrified about the possible damage that she had done. However, she didn't feel like she could stop. She was eating irregularly and only allowed herself to eat a meal if she had been able to have a bowel movement that day. Her anxiety was wrapped up in her body image, her appearance, and the possibility of gaining weight. Despite her fears, she was willing to take the necessary steps toward healing.

Did any parts of those stories sound familiar to you? Even if their particular disordered behavior is not a problem for you, maybe other parts of their stories resonated with you. Maybe you have shared some thoughts, feelings, and struggles with the patients listed above.

Regardless of how much you found in common with those stories, telling your story and unpacking how disorder manifested in your life will help you begin to put things in order. So, take some time to think about your behaviors that need to be examined and changed. In the chapters ahead, we will talk about specific ways to change these behaviors.

Prayer

Lord, please show me how my relationship with food and body is disordered. What things have my family culture, me, or society normalized that are not healthy? Bring clarity and insight into my mind and spirit and let me see what needs to change. Give me hope as I begin to realize my emotions are valid, but my behaviors may not be serving me anymore. Help me Jesus to have eyes to see, ears to hear, and a heart to know your truth. In Jesus' name, Amen.

Invitation

In your journal, begin to detail what disordered behaviors have crept in over the years and where they started. If new memories come up for you, write those down too in as much detail as you can so you can remember your feelings around these memories. It may be very uncomfortable to remember these events in your life. That discomfort is not in vain. Detailing your disordered behaviors can help you recognize your emotions, thoughts, and beliefs about food and your body both past and present. This will help you immensely as you learn more in the following chapters about how to create peace with food and your body.

CHAPTER 3

Internal Family Systems

> For I know that through your prayers and God's provision of the Spirit of Jesus Christ, what has happened to me will turn out for my deliverance.
>
> —Philippians 1:19

Internal Family Systems (IFS) is a therapeutic model that was created in the 1990s by Richard C. Schwartz (IFS Institute). IFS recognizes that our souls have different parts, and we can strategically lead those parts away from well-meaning but destructive behaviors and back to their useful and life-giving purposes (Schwartz, 2019).

I will not attempt to describe IFS in more detail in this book, but I highly recommend that you study it further on your own. I wanted to mention it because it is the most effective therapeutic framework I have found in my practice as an eating disorder dietitian.

In my earlier years of practice, I would tell patients that their eating disorder was abusive or harmful, likening it to an abusive relationship. I would tell them they had to "stop these behaviors for good" and use other language that was too harsh. I constantly gave my clients the impression that their eating disorders needed to be banished from their lives and that their behaviors were just downright evil.

Throughout the years, IFS has taught me that disordered eating and body image struggles are harmful in the way they are manifested, but often these behaviors seem to be the best way we can find to protect ourselves in the moment. In other words, *the intent of the disorder is oftentimes very, very good. It is the manifestation we need to adjust.* The intent should be appreciated and redirected.

What is the Intent Behind Your Disorder?

I recently presented this therapeutic framework (IFS) to a client who used restrictive behaviors to keep her weight low (below what would normally be healthy for her). She had suffered from sexual and physical abuse in the past, and restriction afforded her a sense of control and protection against further abuse. She believed that if she kept her weight down, not only would she experience less pain about her past trauma, but she would also be less attractive to men who may try to abuse her in the future. *Food restriction was her protector.*

Using IFS to reframe maladaptive behaviors with food and body is much more respectful to patients than demanding change. Using this perspective, I would never demand that safety, protection, or control be taken away from you, even if it is only perceived.

For this particular client, I asked her to thank the restriction for what it had done for her up to this point. I asked her to appreciate how many times it had allowed her to perceive herself as safe. Then I asked her to consider what eating behaviors would *actually* keep her safe.

We then explored the idea that being well-nourished results in physical strength, mental agility, and emotional stability. She was able to understand that food provided more protection than restriction did. We acknowledged that if she ever felt really scared or really out of control in this process, she could always go back to her restriction. This was groundbreaking for her. She was eventually able to trust the security of food and energy more than the false security of restriction and anorexia nervosa.

In this journey of discovering what is out of order and trying to achieve peace with food, movement, rest, and body image, I would like for you to keep the theory of IFS at the forefront of your mind. As you recognize what behaviors need to be changed around food, movement, rest, and body image, also recognize how your maladaptive behaviors have served you, protected you, and helped you cope with your life. Thanking the disordered behaviors for all they have afforded you in the past will bring comfort to that part of your soul.

Remember that, although I hope and pray for your total peace and freedom, you can always go back to the disorder. You have that freedom, and if your knees are knocking, I hope that reassurance will help you. I would never demand that you leave behind behaviors that have helped you survive. I only hope to offer you new ones to help you thrive.

Sometimes the truth comes swiftly, and sometimes it comes gently. Internal Family Systems can be a gentler way to approach recovery, especially if you have suffered trauma. In this approach, I hope you find peaceful validation and an invitation to try something different. What if those well-meaning parts of your soul that led you to the disorder could take a back seat? They don't have to leave completely. What if you can meet your needs in healthier ways? What if you could be at peace with food, movement, rest, your body, and inside your very soul?

Prayer

Lord, please reveal how well-meaning parts of me have used destructive behaviors to cope with the pain of my life. Please show me my unhealthy coping mechanisms and give me courage to change. Help me, Lord, to understand how to embrace my pain, comfort those aching parts of me, but not let them lead me. Please help me to be led by your spirit instead of my pain. Help me to begin to learn how to get my needs met in healthy, fulfilling ways. God, be with me as I keep going, and please do what only You can do. In Jesus's name, Amen!

Invitation

If you would like to, take some time to write in your journal about how your disorder with food, movement, rest, or body image has helped you survive parts of your life. Acknowledge that although your behaviors may have been unhealthy, the intent behind them was good. Thank your unhealthy behaviors for all they have done for you and let those parts of you - the angry, the anxious, the fearful, the sad parts of you - which led you to use unhealthy behaviors know you are going to be trying a new approach. In the pages that follow you will be given a new approach to get your good, normal, God-given needs met.

CHAPTER 4

Healing a Past of Brokenness

Then you will know the truth, and the truth will set you free.

—John 8:32

A long time ago, while listening to a sermon, I heard a phrase that hit me right between the eyes. The pastor was speaking about matters that often come up in every family. In this context, he said, "There is no pain greater than family pain, and there is no joy greater than family joy." Those words traveled to the marrow of my bones that day, and there they have stayed. Our greatest sorrows and our greatest joys often do come through family members and the sometimes complicated relationships we have with them.

With eating disorders or any sort of issue with food and the body, there is no single culprit. In fact, wisdom tells us there is never one source of blame in any situation. There are always a host of circumstances, people, and precipitating factors that lead to disorder and a loss of health. Still, there are a few very common denominators in every story, and one of them is family. Whether you have a diagnosable eating disorder, a mild disruption with healthy behaviors, or anything in between, somewhere within the layers of events, reasons, and root causes, you will find at least one family member.

A Word About Honesty

A few years ago, I was scrolling through Instagram when I came across a post by faith leader Havilah Cunnington. All it said was, "Liars don't heal" (Cunnington). She's right. One cause of staying stuck in dysfunction of any kind is the unwillingness to accept the truth of a situation. In other words, denial and pretending might protect us from pain, but they also hold us back from living our most meaningful lives. Only acceptance and a desire to change can help us heal from our wounds.

If you find yourself feeling uncomfortable with the idea of analyzing how your family has influenced you in the areas of food, movement, rest, and body image, I understand. Remember my pastor's quote from earlier? "There is no pain like family pain." I have been treating beautiful souls with disordered eating for fifteen years, and I have seen the miraculous healing of God in so many lives. Seeing God's work keeps me going even though it's difficult to hear the pain in my clients' stories. It's also why I wrote this book.

I want you to heal, but in order to do that, you have to be honest with yourself. You have to go to the dark places of your story so you can bring light into them. For some, family trauma might be so severe that it should only be explored within the safety of formal treatment. Whether the pain associated with your family is little or extreme, my prayer for you is to be honest with yourself about your story so you can receive healing.

If you are willing to risk looking at how your family may have hurt you in the areas of food, movement, rest, and body image, then you are opening yourself up to receive lasting change. This change will heal you and others in your circle of influence and your family line.

Measuring Your Worth

In looking at how our families may have impacted us and our relationships with food, movement, rest, and body image, first, I will address the scale. Cultural norms about body size and weight are different across the world. But no matter what culture we come from, our familial norms about body size and weight will influence our thoughts more than anything else.

How often are you weighing yourself? What emotions do you experience after you see the number on your scale? When your body changes, for better or worse, do you ever think about what family members will say about those changes? Was weight a common topic of discussion amongst your family members when you were growing up? Is it still a common topic?

Family members might not specifically discuss your weight, but maybe they constantly criticize their own or other peoples' bodies. The way in which a person speaks about weight or appearance is indicative of how much that person values weight and appearance. Comments made about your body are not a judgment of your worth; rather, they are an indication of the speaker's values and biases. Unfortunately, we often assign judgments to ourselves well before we are able to understand this truth. Consequently, the scars run deep.

Our society sees weight as a way to measure someone's worth rather than just a way to measure the mass of someone's body. Clearly, there are some big problems with this. Namely, it is very damaging to use a data point of any kind to label value, pass judgment, or influence someone's self-esteem. Weight, like many other measurements of our bodies, is a variable with many precipitating factors. Diet and exercise are far from the only things that can impact a person's weight.

God created each body so differently. No two are the same, and yet we sit under immense pressure to look similar to each other. Have you ever thought about why we feel this pressure? You might think, "Well, because I want to be healthy, and I want to make sure I take care of my body." That is usually one of the first reasons I hear when I ask someone about their goals while working with me. I also hear things like, "I just want to be okay in my body, "I don't want to hate it anymore," "I want to stop fighting my body," and "I am so tired of constantly feeling like I need to lose weight."

As a healthcare provider, I would hope that each of us is concerned with our health. I would like to think that everyone is mindful of their individual health concerns and genetic predispositions, and understand the basics of nutrition and exercise science. But all too often, when I hear people talk about their weight issues, no one is actually talking about health.

What is Your Real Motivation?

As humans, we are naturally impatient. We might know that slow, gradual changes are the key to lasting health improvement, but the desire for quick change indicates a motivation other than health improvement. There is an immediate need, and it is not to find out that all of our labs were within normal limits this year. So, could it be that when we say we want to lose weight or look a certain way, we actually desire something much, much deeper and more significant? Clearly, I would say yes.

Above our desire to see our health markers fall into place, there is usually a greater desire for the scale to say a certain number. We think, "If I could get to that number, I would… fill in the blank." I would be able to fit into those clothes again. I would feel so much better about myself. I would look like I used to. I would finally be comfortable in my body again. I would feel attractive. I would get the attention I need. I would get the approval I need. I would get the love I need.

Can you see the direct correlation between weight and meeting some of our most important core needs as human beings? How did this happen? Why did we start putting so much value on what we weigh and, ultimately, what we look like? Again, I believe the culture within our families is one of the biggest influences on this.

But why? Why is family so important to all of us? Two of the biggest needs of humans are *belonging* and *significance*. These needs were first introduced by early psychology leader Alfred Adler as the primary needs of every child (Adler, n.d.). If in childhood these needs are not met, or if they are only met if the child looks a certain way, the consequences can be devastating. For many people, the feeling of significance or belonging in their family is either partly or fully dependent on their outward appearance. Because of this, they do everything they can to look a certain way or weigh a certain weight. It is exhausting to live under that immense pressure.

I believe it is time to release the pressure. Our bodies were never meant to meet our needs for belonging and significance. Author Curt Thompson writes, "We all are born into the world looking for someone looking for us, and that we remain in this mode of searching for the rest of our lives" (Thompson, 2021). What does this mean? We all need to feel valued, loved, cared for, liked, enjoyed, and special. If we receive the message that these needs will only be met if we look a certain way, then it makes a lot of sense why we desire to have a certain body type.

If we think of our bodies as broken cisterns that can never satisfy the need for belonging and significance, then maybe we can release the pressure and stop striving so hard to look a certain way. We need to lovingly detach from the lie that our bodies can provide true significance and belonging. Then, we can focus on what our bodies truly need. We can eat intuitively. We can enjoy food and honor our bodies' cues. We can take health issues into consideration when eating and exercising. And most importantly, we can go to The Source that will actually fulfill us instead of putting all that pressure on our bodies.

Prayer

Lord, family issues are complicated and painful sometimes. I don't want to blame any one person for my issues with food and body, but I want to take an honest look at the messages I received from loved ones about food and my body. I want to uncover what important needs are linked to my weight and body size and what I eat. I want to be able to release the immense pressure I sometimes feel to look a certain way. Please help me go to the root of the issue, my need for love and acceptance. Help me, Jesus, to tell my story, recall my memories I have with family members, and through telling my story, get to a place of forgiveness and peace. In Jesus' name, Amen.

Invitation

If you would like to, get your journal out again and begin to write more of your story. Think about when you were a very small child. Think about how food and body was spoken of in your home. Think of influential times when you remember consciously or subconsciously learning your worth and value was somehow tied to what you ate or what you looked like. Think about how that began to impact you. Ask the Holy Spirit to reveal the lies you began to believe. Try to recognize how these lies are still affecting you today. This work is deep and it can be very painful so please process all of this with trusted loved ones or hire a therapist when needed. Don't forget to take breaks too. Just don't stop. We are just getting started!

CHAPTER 5

Beauty for Ashes: The Ultimate Trade

The Spirit of the Sovereign Lord is on me, because the Lord has anointed me to proclaim good news to the poor. He has sent me to bind up the brokenhearted, to proclaim freedom for the captives and release from darkness for the prisoners, to proclaim the year of the Lord's favor and the day of vengeance of our God, to comfort all who mourn, and provide for those who grieve in Zion—to bestow on them a crown of beauty instead of ashes, the oil of joy instead of mourning, and a garment of praise instead of a spirit of despair. They will be called oaks of righteousness, a planting of the Lord for the display of his splendor.

—Isaiah 61:1–3

In the last chapter, we started to dip our toes in some pretty deep waters. We started to process how our families have helped create the dysfunctional ways we behave toward food and our bodies. It is hard to remember painful memories and even harder sometimes to let ourselves tell the full truth about our stories. For most of us, there are very deep rooted beliefs that say "if I looked a certain way, I would get my most important needs met. My pain would lessen or even cease and

I would finally be at peace." If we look at our dysfunctional behaviors through that lens, all of the dieting, the overexercise, and the plastic surgery makes sense.

But there is another way…

It's time to exchange the immense pressure that has been placed on our bodies for the deep, unconditional significance and belonging that we can experience through Jesus Christ. We can trade worrying about our weight or trying to look a certain way for a restoration of truth and childlike assurance. This kind of assurance promises belonging and significance, no matter what our past looks like (or what our bodies look like). I believe God wants to give you peace with your body and peace with your past.

In order to have the peace we long for, we have to take an honest look at the messages we received from others and how we have supported self-oppression. We have to:

1. Acknowledge the dysfunction that was put on us by sometimes very well-meaning family members
2. Challenge the dysfunction
3. Decide what we are going to claim as truth
4. Forgive the person who has harmed us

We have to repeat this sequence over and over, as many times as it takes, until the bitterness subsides and we are left with peace. Over time, the dysfunction will transform into a testimony of how truth and forgiveness can change anything in our lives.

To help you better understand the idea of "what we were given by others and how we have supported self-oppression," here are a few examples of clients who came to understand this subject better:

Jenny's Story

When Jenny started unpacking her family's influence on her self-esteem and eating habits, she recalled a specific moment that haunted her. When she was ten years old, she overheard her father say to her mother, "If [Jenny] can keep her weight down, she will have it all. She will have everything going for her." Jenny told me, "Kristen, I wasn't overweight at all. I was normal. I was even thin, I think. That was just my natural body. And I never thought anything about weight.

"My mom had always struggled with her weight and made terrible comments about how fat and disgusting she was, but I had never thought much about my weight until that moment. I realized if I ever came close to being overweight, I might lose my parents' favor. That day the approval of my parents, which is so lofty for any child, became tied to my weight, and I have carried that ever since."

Rachel's Story

Another client, Rachel, told me she was speaking to one of her favorite family members one day. This woman was older than her and was someone she loved and cared for deeply. Rachel asked this loved one about her daughter and how she was doing. The loved one answered, "She is okay, but my goodness, she is getting big. I am just worried if she doesn't get that weight off, she is never going to." Rachel, unfortunately, wasn't shocked by this statement.

She reported, "As much as I can rely on this family member for emotional support and to speak truth to me, in this area, she just doesn't get it. She thinks and feels that her worth and value lie in her body size, and she projects that onto all the other girls in our family. I know this, so I don't even talk to her about it, which is really sad. I wish I could be honest with her about how much it has hurt me over the years and how useless this conversation feels."

Gabrielle's Story

After years of gastrointestinal issues as a result of her malnutrition and eating disorder, Gabrielle's body had finally healed. She was able to eat a much bigger variety of foods that were high in fiber and rich in flavor. On one occasion, shortly after she realized she could eat a much bigger variety in her recovery, she went out to eat with her mother.

She ordered a salad with all the toppings. She said, "It was amazing. It was so delicious, and I could have cried. I was so happy to be able to eat something like that and know I was not going to be in terrible pain when I was done. My mom's reaction as I ate, and ate quickly because it tasted so good, was to make pig noises at me and to tell me I should probably slow down. I was devastated. All of the joy I felt over that success and my healing was stolen when she made that comment."

Did any of those family interactions sound familiar to you? Many of you will have memories, both cherished and painful, that come to mind as you work through these pages to be at peace with food and your body. Don't take these memories lightly. Your story, memories, and pain will guide you to the places that need healing most.

Prayer

Lord, thank You for my family. They are beautiful and broken, just as I am. Please reveal to me the people and events that shaped my beliefs and fears surrounding food and my body. Please help me recognize the places that need the most healing from you. Give me the courage, oh God, to know I can heal with Your help. Help me to see what needs to be seen, leave what needs to be left, take what needs to come with me, and forgive along the way. Give me beauty for ashes and joy for my mourning. Thank You, God, for the space and time to do this beautiful, hard, important work. In Jesus's name, Amen.

Invitation

If you would like to, keep writing in your journal about the specific messages you were given by your family members related to food and body image. What conversations were had around weight, body image, movement, rest, and food? How did your parents or caretakers show you that you belonged in your family and that you were significant to them? You can write stories in great detail or just jot memories down.

You might have difficulty remembering parts of your childhood that would unlock some of what was given to you. Don't worry about that right now. Just ponder how your family and loved ones have affected you in the areas of food, movement, rest, and body image.

If you take the time to explore this and commit to being honest with your answers, the pressure release will come. The insight into how those events still affect you and your behaviors today will also come. They may come quickly, or they may come slowly, but they will come. When you are ready, I will see you in part two!

PART II

Peace with Food

CHAPTER 1

How to Start Having Peace With Food

Commit to the Lord whatever you do, and He will establish your plans.

—Proverbs 16:3

Many years ago, I worked at an inpatient treatment facility for women with eating disorders. I led a group session every week called Bulimic Group. The group was created to give patients the chance to engage with commonly binged foods in a safe, mindful way. We would fill the space with foods that contained high levels of dietary fat and carbohydrates. We would then help the patients portion the foods and create snacks that were nutritionally appropriate.

At one particular Bulimic Group session, we presented the patients with many varieties of potato chips and a display of assorted doughnuts. We started the session by asking everyone how they were feeling about being there that day. We also asked the patients to share what their personal intentions and goals were for the session.

When it was her turn to speak, one patient took a deep breath and announced with all the confidence and joy that she could muster, "Today is the day I will shake hands with a doughnut!" After many giggles and clapping all around, she explained further: "I have binged so many times on doughnuts. I have eaten way too many at a time, felt so much shame, and betrayed myself and my health countless times while eating doughnuts. But it was never really about the doughnuts. Now that I have realized this, I can eat one. Just one. I will enjoy it and be satisfied." With so much clarity and joy, she was able to overcome her fear and take a step forward.

What Does Peace With Food Mean?

Peace with food means putting food in its proper place in your life. It happens when you don't idolize or demonize food but allow yourself to enjoy it. Peace with food involves making a plan for what you will eat every day and every week. It also involves plenty of flexibility, because life happens and plans change. It is thinking about food as a part of your routine and taking the time to make sure your nutritional needs are met each day.

Peace with food means taking health issues, allergies, etc., into consideration but also having the freedom to deviate from your plan when necessary. It means being confident in knowing general healthy practices around food and not relying on food to meet any other needs outside of hunger. It involves using coping mechanisms besides food to handle your emotions.

What does "peace with food" mean to you? I know for my patient mentioned above, it meant the war was over. She decided that day not to use food to cope with hard things in her life anymore. That day she separated food from her most deeply rooted needs. She stopped relying on food for comfort and stopped looking to her body, shape, size, and weight to fulfill her innermost desire for approval.

By "shaking hands" with a doughnut that day, she was saying, "I am going to face my problems using coping skills that can bring *actual* healing, protection, comfort, and relief." Remember, disordered eating does not meet your needs long term. Your disordered behaviors might have worked for a short time to fix the following problems:

- They might have been a distraction (dieting and following rules)
- They might have helped you feel like you are in control (restriction, purging, excessive exercise)
- They might have helped you meet good and healthy needs (attention, affirmation, acceptance)

However, I would venture to say if you are now on part two of this book, those behaviors may not be working for you quite as well anymore. Peace with food is possible. It will take time and a lot of hard work, but it is possible. Remember the junk drawer from part one? It's time to put a few more things in their proper place.

So far, we have explored our thoughts, feelings, and behaviors and how those were influenced by others. Now we will explore what our bodies need nutritionally. We can meet our bodies' nutritional needs without living in fear or guilt. I want to empower you in this part to better listen to your body and give it what it needs. When you put new perspectives and habits in place, peace will permeate your relationship with food.

It's Only a Matter of Time

Patience isn't exactly one of my strong suits, and I have always despised the saying, "It's only a matter of time." When I hear this, all I can think is, "Yeah, I know, and it is going to take forever." As I have gotten older, I have come to the conclusion that things worth doing usually take longer than we would like them to. We usually appreciate things more when it takes a long time for us to get them.

It's not that we don't have the time to put forth the effort; we just don't often want to. I promised you in the introduction of this book that this process of finding true peace with food, movement, rest, and body image was going to take longer than you would like. I feel the need to remind you of this again.

One of the lures of diet culture is how fast everything seems to happen. Diets promise better health and confidence, and there is always a timeline associated with it. Sometimes it only takes as little as two weeks, thirty days, sixty days, or ninety days to get to "a better you," "a beach body," or "your ideal weight." They claim that a fast delivery of weight loss will fix all your problems. *When we are in physical or emotional pain, that sounds like such a great solution.*

Let it Go

Before we go any further in regards to finding true peace with food, I am going to ask you to let go of a few things. Let go of your timeline, your scale, and those pants in the back of your closet that you are using as a measuring stick. You know the pants I am talking about. Throw them out. Literally.

Please hear me: goals are good. I love goals, and I want you to set them. But if you have struggled with food for even five minutes, your soul has probably been injured by shame in this area. Shame tells us we are good for nothing. Shame doesn't just tell us that we have done something wrong; it tells us that we *are* wrong.

If you have shame about food or your body, the best way to challenge your shame is to drag it into the light. If you are still struggling with a strong diet mentality and you find yourself wanting to be smaller, change your body in some way, or fit into certain pants again, be honest about it. Change your perspective by *giving yourself all the time you need* to put things in order with your relationship with food.

If you continue to put pressure on yourself to "be done" by a certain time, you are going to have a much harder time making the progress you want to make in this area. Fortunately, chances are, it won't take years and years. So, take a deep breath and give yourself over to this process, *no matter how long it takes.*

My Nutrition Philosophy

We all have beliefs about food which are ingrained into our minds and come out through our actions. I have already encouraged you to start digging into your story so you can find out where your beliefs come from. As I guide you on your journey of creating peace with food, my hope is your philosophy about food and your body will be aligned with the truth of how God created your body.

My nutrition philosophy has gone through an overhaul since getting my degree in 2008. Unfortunately, much of what I received in my upbringing and in my education was steeped heavily in diet culture. Working with clients with eating disorders for 15 years has helped me heal and made me realize the truth about food.

My nutrition philosophy is very simple. We were created to eat and enjoy food. There are no good or bad foods. There is no morality attached to what foods we choose to eat. Not all foods are created equal, but all foods fit into a healthy diet when eaten in balance, variety, and moderation. No foods are off-limits.

Food is to be used for fuel, but also for pleasure and even comfort at times. Food was given to us by design by a loving God who created us to need it and enjoy it. Therefore, it should be enjoyed. The key to healing our relationship with food is to stop trying so hard to follow a strict set of rules and to discover the motivation behind why we eat the way we do. When we eat according to what our bodies are telling us we need, we can have lasting peace.

Prayer

Lord, all of this letting go of pressure and allowing for flexibility seems very foreign to me. Help me continue on this journey to find peace. Give me courage, God. Where I have relied on rigidity and rules around food, give me freedom and knowledge. Help me to let go of the false sense of control dieting has given me in the past. Help me begin to see how honoring my body and listening to its cues gives me actual control. Help me put my relationship with food in order so I can have peace. In Jesus' name, Amen.

Invitation

In your journal, continue to unpack areas where you currently do not feel peace with food. Use this time to identify your personal philosophy about food and where it might need to be challenged and changed. Be honest about your current behaviors with food and evaluate if they are based on fear and diet culture. If so, take some time to make goals you would like to put in place for how you relate to food. Define what peace with food would look like to you in the weeks and months to come. In other words, ask God for a vision of how a peaceful relationship with food would look like for you.

CHAPTER 2

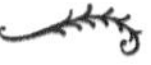

Food Education: Meals, Snacks, and Water

The boundary lines have fallen for me in pleasant places;
surely I have a delightful inheritance.

—Psalm 16:6

When teaching the process of how to make peace with food, there is a wealth of nutrition information that could be shared. For the purposes of this book, I am only going to list the most practical habits and useful facts about nutrition. If you are looking for a more in-depth study of the body and nutrition, I trust you will find a plethora of wonderful resources to take you further than we have time for in this book. I pray you will take what is pertinent to you from this list and apply it right away.

Breakfast

"All good things start with breakfast." "Breakfast is the most important meal of the day." I know these phrases are cliché, but they are also true. Intermittent fasting is a very popular diet trend right now, but it's not the first one that has tried to limit the amount of time in a day that our body has to meet its hunger needs. Diet peddlers are trying to convince you and me that they know better than our Creator about when we need to feed these amazing bodies of ours.

Most of the time, when a new client comes to me, they are not eating breakfast. So many of the maladaptive behaviors they experience stem from this unwise decision. When you wake up, the clock starts ticking; your energy requirements increase, and *you need to make a plan to make sure you get a balanced breakfast in your body within one hour of waking.*

Eating breakfast accomplishes several things. Most importantly, it sends a clear message to your body that you are going to listen to it and honor its need for energy (calories) that day. And after this becomes a habit, you will no longer experience aversion to food or a lack of hunger in the morning, which is common for those who omit breakfast. After two or three weeks (or less) of eating breakfast consistently, any symptoms of nausea or disinterest in food will be replaced with a delightful craving for a balanced meal in the morning.

If you have to wake up extremely early for work or exercise frequently in the morning after waking up, it may be more realistic to give yourself a two-hour window of time to eat after waking. That is okay, too, and will serve a similar purpose for getting your day started well. Whenever possible, try to eat breakfast within one hour of rising.

But Kristen! If I eat breakfast, I am probably going to be hungrier throughout the day and will eat more calories. And what if that leads to more weight gain? I am trying to be healthier, not gain weight I will have to take off later! If I just read your mind, I wish I could give you a hug right now. Get all your fears out about every step I am recommending. Wrestle with them and come to a place where you can go forward.

Also, I am going to remind you of a few truths:

- Your health is dictated by much more than the number on the scale.
- If you gain weight in this process of making peace with food, your healthy body weight might be higher than you previously thought (especially if you started this process underweight).

- You may notice temporary weight increases along the way because your body needs time to trust that you are not taking it through another feast-and-famine cycle of eating.
- You may not know what will happen to your weight during this process, but you will be healthier overall if you are nourishing your body more consistently and listening to it.
- Peace with food is not about achieving a certain weight. It is about getting your needs met even if your weight is higher than you would like it to be. It is about feeling loved, lovable, attractive, and confident no matter what the number is on the scale.

Until you learn how to take care of your body and give it the time it needs to settle into a comfortable weight range (if it is not already there), you will continue to live in fear of food. You have to be willing to keep your "ideal weight" in an open hand. In other words, you have to take a risk if you want to see change. You have to let go of trying to control your body.

I know - this is harder than you thought it would be. Take some time to write about it in your journal. Try to write down all of your thoughts and fears before you read on. Then, when you are ready, let's talk about meals and snacks!

Meals and Snacks

Every individual body is different, and nutrition needs are going to vary to some degree. That being said, we do know that *most adults are going to need three full meals and one to three snacks each day* in order to meet their nutrition and energy needs. This means that if you are eating breakfast within an hour of waking, you should be eating every two and a half to four hours on average throughout the day. If there are more than four hours between meals and snacks, your blood sugar is likely to get too low.

If you are coming from a restrictive background, you might be thinking, *That is way too much food, and there is no way I need that much*. Well, you actually do need more food than you are used to eating, and eventually, you will feel your body's relief that you are feeding it properly.

What is a Meal?

Put simply, *a meal is an entrée plus one or two sides*. An entrée is one to one and a half cups of a combination food like a casserole or a mixture of protein, fat, and carbohydrates. Here are some examples of entrees:

- Whole sandwiches
- Whole wraps made with at least ten-inch tortillas
- Two or three tacos in shells
- Three to five ounces of chicken, beef, or fish

Sides might consist of:

- One cup of vegetables
- Half a cup of fruit
- Six ounces of yogurt
- A one-ounce bag or a very open handful of chips, pretzels, etc.
- A whole medium-sized piece of fruit
- A medium-size cookie
- Eight ounces of a caloric beverage of any kind

Using these guidelines, a full meal could look like:

- Five ounces of fish with one cup of rice and one cup of cooked vegetables
- Three chicken tacos with half a cup of rice and half a cup of beans
- A whole sandwich made with two to three ounces of meat and condiments with an apple

- A salad with two cups of chopped vegetables and lettuce with three ounces of chicken, shredded cheese, a sprinkle of nuts, and dried fruit with two to three tablespoons of salad dressing and a one-ounce bag of pretzels or chips

Entree + 1-2 sides = Full Meal	
ENTREE: One to one and a half cups of a combination food like a casserole or a mixture of protein, fat, and carbohydrates	**1-2 SIDES:** What is a side??
1-1.5 c. casserole	1 c. vegetables
1 whole sandwich	1 c. fruit
2-3 tacos with shells	1 medium-size piece of fruit
1 whole sandwich wrap made with at least a 10-inch wrap	6 oz. yogurt
3-5 oz. chicken, beef, or fish	1 medium-size cookie
6-9 sushi rolls	8 oz. of a caloric beverage of any kind
1.5-2 c. soup/stew	1 oz. bag or a very open handful of chips, pretzels, etc.

Snack= should have a combination of foods represented in each snack. The best way to think about this is to think that snacks must be "two parts," meaning one part coming from one food group and the second part coming from a different group.	
SNACK PART 1: **Grain, Fruit, or Vegetable**	**SNACK PART 2:** **Dairy, Protein, or Fat**
Crackers (grain)	Cheese (dairy)
Apple (fruit)	Peanut butter (protein)
Carrots (vegetable)	Ranch Dressing (fat)

What is a Snack?

In most cases, there should be two parts in every snack. Both parts should come from different food groups. Examples include crackers and cheese (grain and dairy), apple and peanut butter (fruit and protein), or carrots and ranch dressing (vegetable and fat).

Fortunately, there are endless combinations of foods we can put together for meals and snacks. Each one of us is going to come up with different versions of what meals and snacks look like in our homes.

There are many things that could impact your eating habits, but guilt, fear, and shame should no longer be factors. Your food preferences should instead be impacted by culture, taste, enjoyment, balance, variety, satisfaction, curiosity, joy, and permission. If the latter list is used to create a new meal plan for yourself, you are going to find your path of eating and nourishment laden with more peace than you have ever known.

Water

Water is essential for life. We know this, but do you know why? Proper hydration affects every mechanism in every single organ of the body. Water is utilized in every single cell. It is the carrier of electrolytes into our cells, and it regulates our blood viscosity. Water affects our ability to absorb and digest nutrients in our gastrointestinal tract. The list goes on and on.

I often hear clients say, "I hate water. It is so boring. I will drink a little bit, but doesn't everything else have water in it? Isn't it enough just to drink liquids?" Technically, yes, every other liquid does contain some amount of water, but those amounts vary. In the end, we need a lot of *actual* water each day to stay healthy and hydrated. You can up the flavor of "boring water" by infusing it with lemon, lime, or orange slices. Sparkling water is another way to make it more interesting to your taste buds.

Caffeine

I also need to address caffeinated beverages because most of us love our coffee, tea, and the like, which are filled to the brim with a little "go get 'em" for the day! These do not count as hydration. In fact, I hate to be the bearer of bad news, but for every ounce of caffeinated beverage you choose to drink, it cancels out an ounce of water. Caffeine is a diuretic, which means it opens up the body to release more fluids than it naturally would.

Let's take this example: If a person's water requirement is ninety-two ounces per day and they drink ninety-two ounces of water plus twelve ounces of a caffeinated beverage, they have actually only consumed eighty ounces of water. When making nutrition goals, this may cause you to decrease your caffeine intake to either equal to or less than the recommended maximum intake of 400 milligrams of caffeine per day. This is roughly 4 cups of coffee. Just because you can drink this much, certainly doesn't mean you should. Considering the importance of hydration and what we just learned in the examples above, hopefully 1-2 cups of coffee each day will suffice for most of us. That leaves plenty of time to drink adequate amounts of water after you have enjoyed your morning coffee (Caffeine, 2022).

We often get stuck thinking we *need* caffeine to get through the day. I would challenge you to work on getting seven to nine hours of sleep a night and following adequate water intake for your body (see below). Caffeinated beverages should be used for enjoyment rather than as a means to "push through" your day. When used in moderate portions, they can add joy to your life. When overused, just like most things, they begin to tax the body.

Goals for hydration

Most nutrition science references will offer general guidelines for hydration needs because our needs are much more complex than just multiplying our weight by a certain number and coming up with a goal.

A general goal for water consumption for adults would be a minimum of two liters (or sixty-four ounces) per day. From there, paying attention to the color of your urine is one of the most common ways to assess if you are getting enough hydration. The goal is to consistently have light- or pale-yellow urine except for the first time you urinate in the morning (that will always be darker, even in well-hydrated people).

Prayer

Lord, help me to take an honest look at how, when, and why I consume food. When I feel fear about making necessary changes, help me to let go of my fear. Give me faith in you, Lord. You made my body and you know more about what it needs to thrive than I do. As I begin to change my behaviors around food and allow myself more freedom, please remind me my worth and value is so much more than my weight and what I eat. Help me to believe that my needs will be met even if my weight changes and there is no righteousness I can attain by eating a certain way. Sustain me, Lord as I learn a better way. In Jesus' name, Amen.

Invitation

If you would like to, journal your thoughts about this chapter and how different your current practices are from what I suggested. Write down fears and concerns you have about changing your practices around food. Make small, sustainable goals to start listening to your body instead of restricting or overeating. Once this small goal is met, make another and keep going!

CHAPTER 3

Food Education: Macronutrients

> So I commend the enjoyment of life, because there is
> nothing better for a person under the sun than to eat
> and drink and be glad. Then joy will accompany them
> in their toil all the days of the life God has given them
> under the sun.
>
> —Ecclesiastes 8:15

Not long ago, one of my clients told me that her sister had started counting calories and macronutrients. I asked her if she wanted to start doing that, and her response was, "No! I feel like if I did that, all I would be doing is counting instead of living." So true! I had trained her well. *Counting instead of living.* There is an alternative to counting, measuring, and agonizing over food choices. We can be mindful without being constantly hypervigilant. We can learn to trust our bodies again, just as we did when we were children (before we had disordered thoughts about food).

God created the human body with the ability to discern what it needs, and He created our minds to comprehend those needs. He gave us all that we need to meet these needs. Going from disorder to order is possible with some intentional effort to do things differently.

We have already talked about breakfast, normal meals, snacks, and the importance of water. Now I would like to empower you with a bit more knowledge and detail about how to balance the nutrients in your meals. I want to educate you so you can have more freedom. I want to encourage more structure with meal planning so you aren't rummaging through your house at mealtimes trying to figure out what you are going to eat.

I am not giving you rules, and I am not telling you what you can and cannot eat. I still stand by my nutrition philosophy. All foods fit into a healthy diet with balance, variety, and moderation. I simply want to make things easier for you and for you to see that you can eat a large variety of foods in a structured way. You can find peace and ease with food, food planning, and food preparation.

I also want to debunk some cultural ideas and myths about our three energy sources: carbs, proteins, and fats. Let's talk about what they are and what they are not. Then we can jump into meal planning and putting food in a practical order.

Carbohydrates

In every nutrition assessment I have ever done, I ask the question, "What are your favorite foods?" If I am speaking to a client who is being honest, they will say, "*Carbs!* I love carbs. Sweet carbs, salty carbs, bread, cake, I just love carbs!" I delight in this answer because we all love carbohydrates (and I love normalizing that for my clients). Some of us love a wonderfully made cupcake, while others look forward to salty carbs like French fries. Some prefer white rice, some love the heartiness of brown rice, while others prefer quinoa or farro. Whatever your preference, we all love carbs because we all love to feel good.

I am not talking about emotional eating here. I am talking about how carbohydrates cause our bodies to physically feel good and operate optimally when they are eaten in balance. We love carbohydrates because that was the way the body was intended to operate. *Carbohydrates are the body's preferred source of energy.*

Therefore, if you eat fewer carbohydrates than needed or none at all, your body cannot supply your cells with enough glucose (carbohydrates in the simplest form). In this case, your body will break down protein or fat instead, but it doesn't like to do that as much. That is not the body's preference. It takes longer for the body to obtain energy from fat or protein. This can result in ketosis (the breakdown of protein for energy), which puts unnecessary stress on the body.

So, what does all of this mean? Your feeling of guilt for loving carbohydrates is like saying you know you shouldn't love to breathe air, but you do! You just can't help yourself! Another example would be to feel guilty for going to the bathroom or covering your body with proper clothing each day.

Energy is a basic, God-given need, and carbohydrates taste so good to everyone because there is a biological pull to have enough at all times. Depriving yourself of them only causes more physiological and mental urgency to have enough. When we don't have permission to eat carbs, our body wants them even more, and this can lead to overeating and bingeing. Carbohydrates are really important, and if you are not allowing yourself to have them, you are damaging your body and your relationship with food. I could write a whole book on this subject alone, but I want to move on and tell you about your body's next energy source.

Protein

Proteins are the building blocks of every single cell of our bodies. They are the foundational form of cellular life. Proteins are made of amino acids. In the diet industry, protein is touted as the best macronutrient to aid in weight loss. That claim is solely based on the diets that are trending at this moment in time. I want to educate you about why God created protein to show you the bigger picture and to help you understand why we need it.

Have you ever been to a Lego store? Does your child's room look like a Lego store? Complete proteins are like a Lego castle. Amino acids are the building blocks of proteins, so they are like the individual Lego blocks.

For years protein has been a very lucrative moneymaker for the diet industry—and it still is today. It is common for diet trends to focus on protein more than it is necessary. As of right now, when I search for "high-protein diets" on Google, there are 918,000,000 results. Think about that for a moment. There are that many places on Google alone where someone can go to study how to use protein in large amounts to lose weight. Instead of joining the mainstream diet culture, I would love to reframe how you think about protein.

Let's look at six basic facts about protein:

- Muscle tissue is made of protein.
- Amino acids allow for the normal exchange and distribution of fluids to occur in the body and are therefore responsible for keeping fluid balance in check.
- Protein is responsible for the strength of your hair, skin, and nails.
- It can be found in a variety of animal and plant sources and can be very satisfying when balanced with fats and carbohydrates.
- When we have high peaks or low drops in our blood sugar, it causes a lot of discomfort and dysregulation (ask any diabetic). Protein helps to stabilize blood sugar levels and shorten recovery time after blood sugar spikes and dips.
- Having protein present in all meals and snacks will help the body slow digestion, fuel itself efficiently, and overall stay happy throughout the day.

As you can see, protein does give our bodies many benefits. However, it shouldn't be put on a pedestal and made more important than carbohydrates or fat. They all work together to create harmony in your body.

Fat

Similar to protein, dietary fat has somewhat of a misleading reputation. The misconception that dietary fat equals body fat has been around for decades. People used to think, *If I eat food that contains dietary fat, it will turn into body fat.* Dietary fat *can* turn into body fat if eaten in excess, just like protein and carbs can, but this is not the norm or the intention of the body.

The body will only insist on storing energy as fat tissue or creating new muscle tissue when it is overfed or weight gain is necessary. When the body receives dietary fat from something you choose to eat, its intention is to utilize it for the many systems it is built to serve. Dietary fat's primary purpose is not to find a home among your other fat cells but to cause you to feel good and satisfied.

Not to get too technical, but I have to tell you at least a few reasons why dietary fat is so important. There are four vital micronutrients that cannot be absorbed properly without the help of dietary fat. They are also known as the four fat-soluble vitamins (vitamins A, D, E, and K). Each of these micronutrients exists to aid the body in these specific ways:

- Vitamin A helps the body develop and maintain healthy eyesight. It is also required for normal cell growth and development throughout the lifespan. Without proper levels of vitamin A, blindness may occur.
- Vitamin D increases bone density and strengthens calcified bone structure until the body is between twenty-five and thirty years old. Then, Vitamin D serves to maintain healthy calcium intake for the body's bone structure. Without Vitamin D, one's bone structure could be frail, weak, and increasingly painful as the body ages. Vitamin D also helps the body maintain healthy cholesterol levels.

- Vitamin E's main job is to make sure our hair, skin, and nails are strong and healthy. Without vitamin E, we would experience thin and easily breakable nails, ridges on the nail bed, thin, dull, and easily breakable hair, and a lack of protective skin cell layers.
- Vitamin K allows the blood to clot, which is very important for obvious reasons. Even if someone is suffering from medical issues where blood clotting could be life-threatening, vitamin K is still essential in the body and is encouraged to be consumed on a consistent basis.

Clearly, these fat-soluble vitamins are extremely important to a healthy body, but they cannot be utilized properly without sufficient amounts of dietary fat.

Lastly, the most extraordinary fact about dietary fat is that it is directly related to healthy brain function. Most of the "gray matter" surrounding the brain is made of fat cells. So, when the body is deprived of proper dietary fat, it can use the gray matter of the brain as its fat source. That is why moderate to severe malnutrition causes noticeable differences in brain function.

I think it's safe to say that dietary fat has many more advantages than diet culture would have us believe! Dietary fat is a very important part of a well-balanced diet, and gaining the freedom to eat it without guilt will benefit you greatly.

Balance Your Macronutrient Equation

As you try to balance carbohydrates, protein, and fat in each meal and snack, remember that some foods contain more than one macronutrient. This might not be news to you, but if you look at food labels, many foods have a combination of all three macronutrients, with one of them carrying the lion's share of that food's content.

For instance, peanut butter is a good example of a food with varying degrees of each macronutrient. There are sixteen grams of fat, eight grams of carbohydrates, and seven grams of protein in a serving (two tablespoons). Therefore, including peanut butter in any meal or snack will give you a good start on a balanced macronutrient equation. There are many other foods like this. Remember, the more balanced the meal or snack, the better.

Prayer

Lord, thank you for making my body so expertly. Continue to guide me in how I need to reframe my thoughts and beliefs about food. As I change my beliefs and behaviors around food, help me to know when I get fearful of gaining weight, going out of control with food, what people will think, or any of the other scary thoughts that may come up. Help me to stay present, challenge the lies I have believed, and continue to work towards peace with food. In Jesus' name, Amen.

Invitation

If you would like to, get your journal out and catalog the lies you have believed about eating in a balanced way and the truths you would like to try to replace them with. Celebrate the ways in which you are learning about your body and make small goals to do things differently. Try your best to pay attention to the thoughts and beliefs about food that come up in the days to come. Make a point to align yourself with scientific and biblical truth where diet culture has previously reigned.

CHAPTER 4

Food Education: Meal Planning

In their hearts humans plan their course,
but the Lord establishes their steps.

—Proverbs 16:9

Family/Personal Menu

Now that I have covered our three wonderful macronutrients, let's talk about meal planning! When you sit down and try to think of what you should eat in the coming week, sometimes it is hard to remember all of your options. You might ask your family for dinner ideas or requests for the coming week because you are drawing blanks. This is why creating a menu will serve you well in every season of life!

Your family or personal menu will help you quickly remember what you cook, what everyone likes, and what options are good for your meal plan each week. Take a sheet of paper, a note on your phone, a Word document, or an Excel sheet, and begin listing all of the options you or your family enjoy for breakfast, lunch, dinner, and snacks.

If you want to get really organized, you can add other categories like beverages, desserts, birthday favorites, and holiday favorites. It will be a list of favorites and, ultimately, a guide to simplified meal planning. It will be an evolving list. Add to it when you find new recipes, develop new tastes for things, or when other family members discover new options. The table below shows an example of a family and personal menu.

Personal Menu

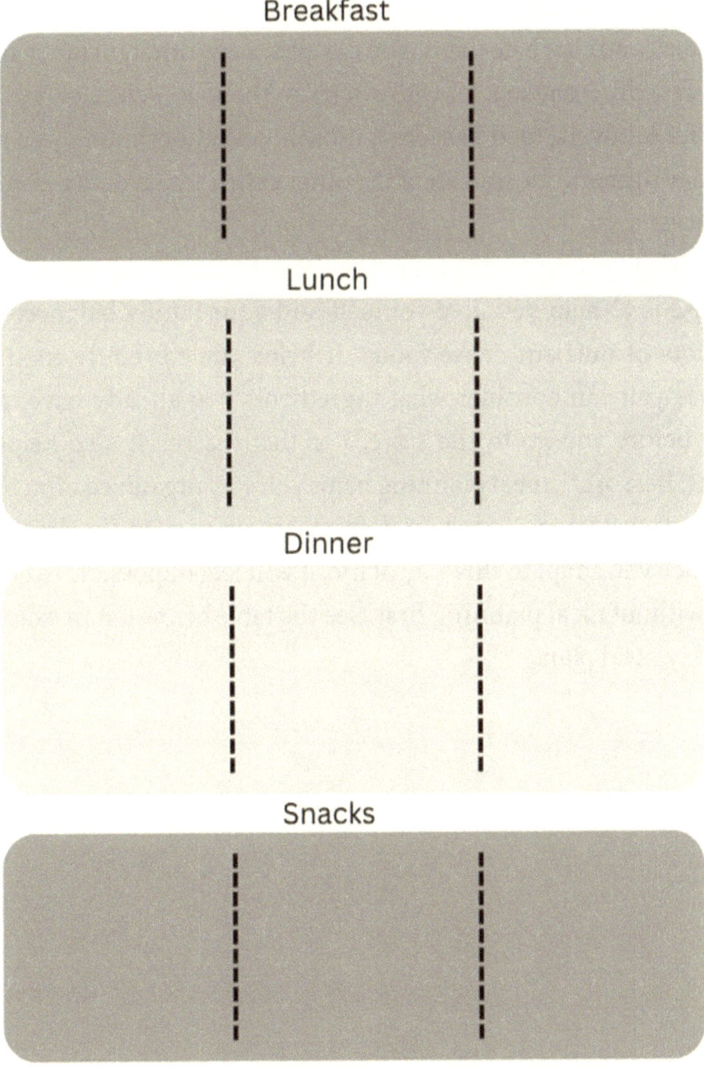

Weekly Meal Plan

The next step in getting your habits with food in order is coming up with a weekly meal plan. Using your family or personal menu for ideas, write down your choices for every day of the week.

Remember, you don't have to pick something different for breakfast, lunch, or snacks every day. You can pick a couple of items for breakfast each week and alternate them. You can pick a few different lunch options and a few different snacks, and alternate them as well. Don't forget to allow for leftovers, taco Tuesdays, monthly neighborhood pizza nights, birthday dinners out, and all of the other eating idiosyncrasies your life produces.

Meal planning is not meant to be a ball and chain for you. Its purpose is to help you give yourself and your family balanced meals with lots of nutrient-dense foods. It helps you to reduce food waste because you can consider what ingredients you already have in your home before you go to the store. For that reason, it also helps your budget. Best of all, meal planning helps you stay organized. You'll know each day what you need to buy, defrost, brown to go in the slow cooker, etc. Once you adapt to this way of life, it will feel impossible to go to the store without meal planning first. See the table below for an example of a weekly meal plan.

Weekly Meal Plan

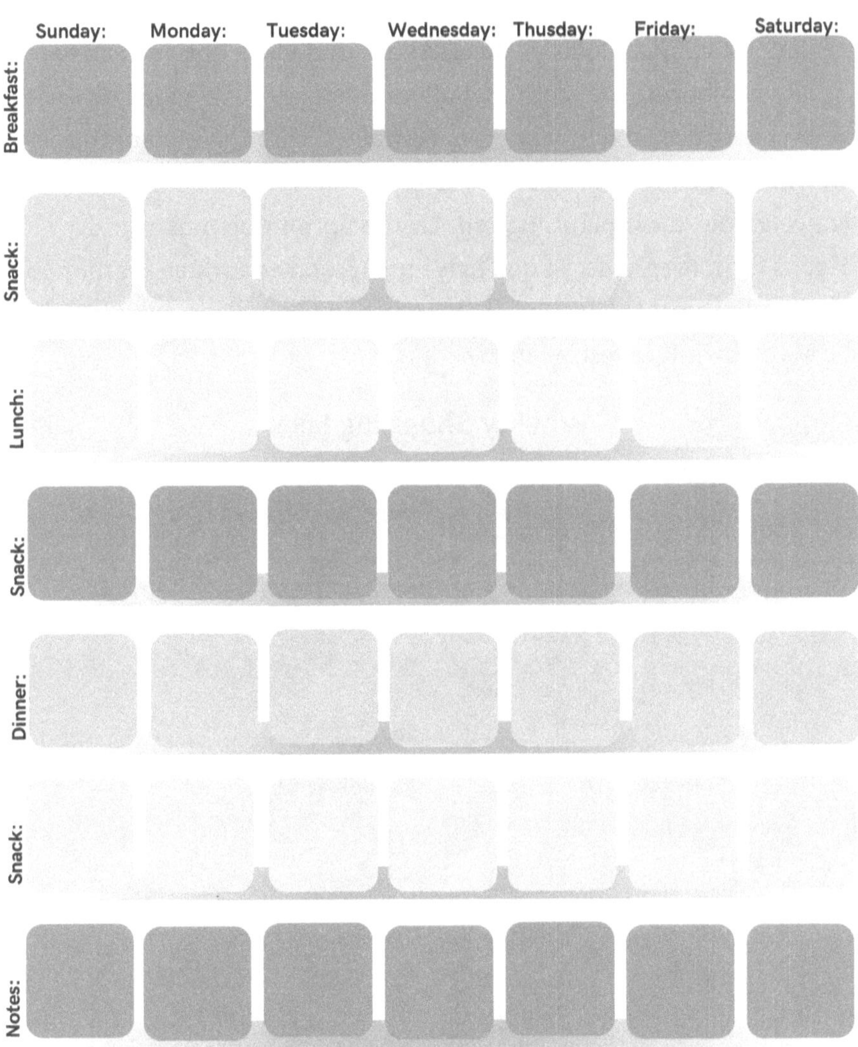

Grocery List

The next step after meal planning is to write your weekly grocery list so you can go shopping. It is always best to go shopping when your belly is full and you are not thinking about food. This helps you to only buy the things you are going to need for the week.

You will be amazed at how much stress, time, and money you'll save when you enter the grocery store with a plan. Below you will find a useful grocery list template to help you plan your next trip to the grocery store.

Remembering the truth that all foods fit into a balanced diet with variety, balance, and moderation, combined with these planning tips, will be a game changer for you. Come back to these truths when life is hectic and meal planning falls to the bottom of your priority list. Habits form over time, so don't give up. If it takes a whole year for you to assimilate meal planning into your life and household culture, it will be a worthwhile investment.

Weekly Shopping List

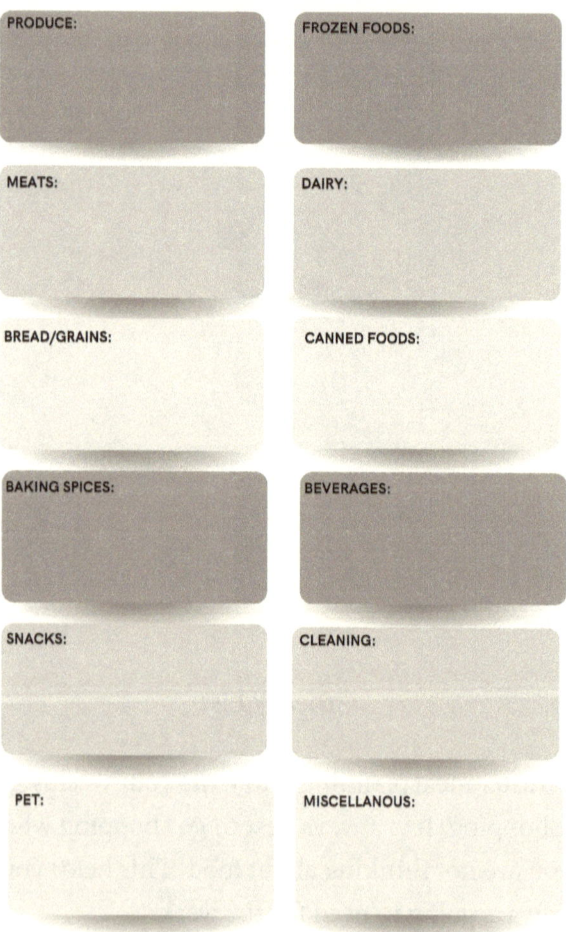

Prayer

Lord, thank you for the ability to create order and the peace that it brings. As I continue to go forward in my journey toward peace and freedom with food, please give me wisdom about what areas need to be more organized. Help me to carve out the time and energy to implement changes that will create peace. Where chaos has been the norm, please help me to lose my tolerance for disorganization. Continue to guide me to your truth in all ways. In Jesus' name, Amen.

Invitation

If you do not already have a personal menu, it is time to make one. This is a great first step because it will help you see how many options you have to feed yourself and your loved ones. Then create a meal plan for just a few days, a week, or even a month. That will guide you in your shopping. All of these steps will greatly aid you in recovering your peace in the area of providing food for yourself. All of the charts in this chapter are listed in the resource list at the back of the book.

CHAPTER 5

Fear Foods

I sought the Lord, and he answered me;
He delivered me from all my fears.Those who look to
him are radiant;
their faces are never covered with shame.

—Psalm 34:4-5

Most people who struggle with eating disorders or disordered eating have what many dietitians refer to as "fear foods" and "safe foods." When fear foods are eaten, they cause the person to feel anxiety, stress, guilt, shame, or even panic at times. Safe foods, on the other hand, cause no anxiety or guilt when eaten. They can be categorized as non-threatening because they are usually low-calorie or "guilt-free."

Sometimes, clients will tell me they don't have any specific fear foods, but they do feel angst about the *quantity* of certain foods they eat. They might say, "I can eat a few doughnut holes, but if I ate an entire doughnut, I would feel really guilty," or, "I can have one or two of my kid's French fries, but if I ate a whole medium-size order of fries, I would be a mess afterward." When hearing this, I gently let my clients know that they do, in fact, have fear foods. Any food that cannot be eaten in a proper portion without having guilt afterward is a fear food to some extent.

Another version of fear foods sounds like this: "I can have sweets, but I can only have them on holidays or special occasions," or, "I can have peanut butter, but then I can't have any other high-fat foods for the rest of the day." That still sounds like fear to me, wouldn't you agree?

For clients who suffer from bingeing or overeating, their fear foods list often looks very similar to their binge foods list. Clients who suffer from restriction and dieting always have a list of fear foods as well.

Do you have a list of fear foods? Pause to write your list in your journal. Think of all the foods that cause you to feel insecure. Think of the foods that you wouldn't dare eat "too much" of for fear of shame and guilt. Take an honest inventory of your fear foods.

Another question to ask yourself when making this list is, "If calories didn't exist and body image issues were foreign to me, what would I start eating that I don't eat currently due to fear?" Did you write your list? Good. You might need to keep adding to it as you go!

How to Interact with Fear Foods

Now, what should you do with that list? Well, if you suffer from bingeing or overeating, the first step is to get rid of all the fear foods in your home. Let me be very clear: this is only temporary, and you are not taking them out of the house because they are "bad" in any way. You are taking them out so you can have new, peaceful interactions with them and separate yourself from the intense feelings that come with bingeing and overeating.

You can't have easy access to your fear foods at first. If they remain in your home while you are trying to heal, it will be a setup for further unwanted interactions with those foods. The length of time they will need to be out of your home will depend on how long it takes you to make peace with those foods. It will also be determined by how willing and able you are to use different coping mechanisms to handle life's difficulties when they arise.

Obviously, if you struggle with buying your fear foods in the first place, you will not need to remove them from your home.

Exposure

The answer to making peace with fear foods is to expose yourself to them in a strategic way. If just thinking about this is making you anxious, don't worry. You are in good company. Every client who I have worked with on fear food exposure is anxious before and during this process. Afterward, however, they are thankful and at peace.

In psychology, one method to overcoming fears is called *exposure with response prevention*. According to this method, in order to work through your fears, you have to face them. You have to do it, even though you are afraid. If you avoid the fear, you are giving away your power. *When you face your fears, you take your power back.* This can be said for any fear you have, including food.

The figure below shows my version of a hierarchy of fear foods. Using this tool, you can take your list of fear foods and categorize them from least to most scary.

Hierarchy of Fear Foods

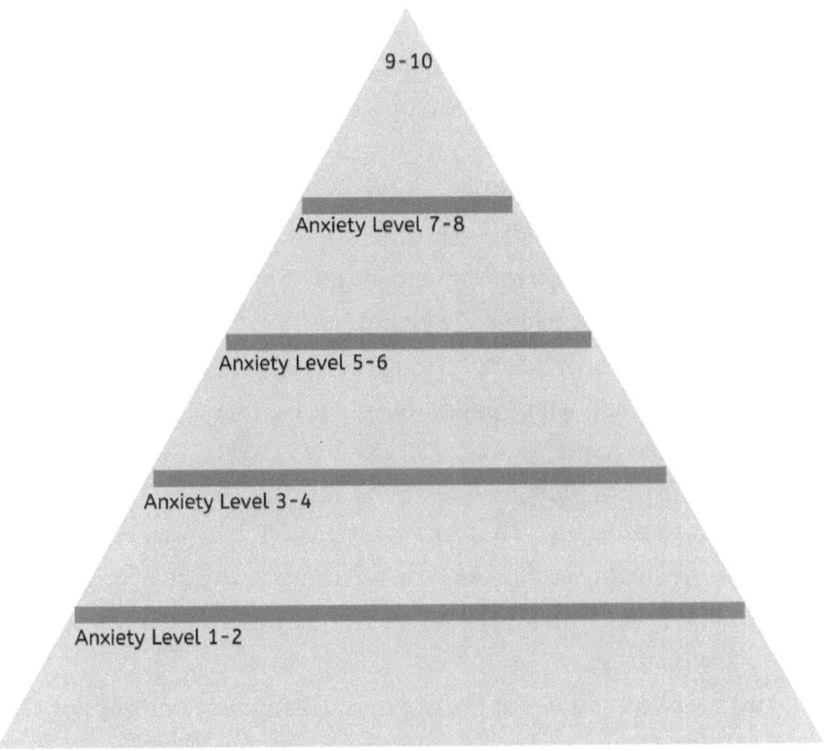

To create a hierarchy of fear foods, begin by listing the foods you are most comfortable with in the bottom tier. Work your way to the top of the pyramid by listing your fear foods with increasing levels of anxiety or fear you feel either before, during, after eating them, or all three.

After categorizing them, I recommend choosing two or three fear foods each week and eating them at least two times that week. Eat them within the context of a normal eating schedule in order to normalize and neutralize the fear of that particular food. In other words, build them into your meal plan. Eating them on purpose and in appropriate portions will feel very scary at first, but it will help you take your power back from these foods and you will begin to feel in control of yourself again around these foods.

If you have removed binge foods from your home, going out of the house for this exposure work will likely be best in the beginning. Going out for certain binge foods accomplishes several things:

- It removes the "I hear it calling me from the pantry" thoughts.
- It allows others in public to see you eating these foods which helps decrease shame, and it will hopefully involve loved ones eating with you to give your support.
- Eating these foods with others will give you accountability, which is highly recommended (most bingeing and overeating happen when people are alone).
- There will only be one serving involved as opposed to a large bag of chips or a whole gallon of ice cream that would be available to you at home.

If you are thinking, *That sounds like a long, expensive process of eating out frequently each week*, you are right. It will be a long process to encounter peace with all of your fear foods, but it probably won't take as long as you think.

You are also right about the expense. Eating out is more expensive than eating at home; however, the effects of disordered eating will cost you way more in the long run. Hiring professionals to help and/or paying for health complications from these behaviors can get *very* expensive. Doing the work of exposure at a pace with which you are comfortable will pay off in the end. Facing your fears and living to tell about them is the only way to the other side. It's the only way to peace.

Bringing certain foods back into your home can happen slowly but surely, too, as you do the exposure work. You will know you have reached peace with each food when you can eat it without feeling intense urges for more after your body is satisfied. Bring the food back into your home when you are no longer tempted to compensate with purging, exercise, restriction, etc.

You can consider yourself at peace with the food when you don't feel any guilt or shame after eating it. Another clear sign that you have made peace with a food is not caring to eat it at all when you have the opportunity. In other words, you could take or leave it. You are not affected by its presence, and you feel like you are in control of your actions around that food. That is what peace with food feels like. Peace is waiting for you, no matter how long you have struggled and how fearful you feel. Exposure work works, and the sooner you try it, the sooner you will experience this.

Prayer

Lord, I have believed lies about food for so long and I have given over so much of my power to food and my behaviors around it. As I make my hierarchy of food fears and make a plan to incorporate these foods into my life in a peaceful way, please hold me. When I am afraid, remind me that I can give my fear over to you and you will help me. When I feel out of control, help me to stop, breathe, and invite you in. Help me, Jesus, take small but steady steps towards food freedom. In your name, Amen!

Invitation

You will find a link to the hierarchy of fear foods on the resource list at the back of this book. If you would like to, make your food fear list and categorize these food fears on the hierarchy so you can have a plan of how to begin your exposure work. You will start with the least anxiety-provoking foods and work your way up to the most anxiety-producing foods. There is no timeline, only yours. As long as you continue to make progress, whenever you get there is great!

CHAPTER 6

Permission with Mindfulness

> Peace I leave with you; my peace I give you. I do not give to you as the world gives. Do not let your hearts be troubled and do not be afraid.
>
> —John 14:27

Whew! Did chapters 1-5 in this part feel like a lot? That's because it was! I hope the education provided will be helpful as you adopt new mindsets and behaviors around food. Before ending this part about making peace with food, we have to acknowledge that education without mindfulness can result in too much rigidity or too much fluidity in your relationship with food.

Let me explain it this way: eating proper meals and snacks, making peace with all foods, viewing food as fuel rather than something to avoid, and following a meal plan are all really good. But, once you do all those things, *you still have to listen to your body in the moment.* In every moment that you are eating, it is all about you and your body. No one else, and nothing else matters. Practice listening to your bodily cues. Eat when you are hungry, eat to satisfaction, but stop when you are physiologically satisfied. It can take some time to figure out those boundaries and remember what it feels like when you are hungry, full, and satisfied. Take the needed time. When you start to listen to your body again, it will reteach you how to listen to it. Be a student of your body again. It is the clearest path to understanding what your body needs.

If you are not truly hungry, think about why you are going to food and what your body *actually* needs. If you eat to satisfaction but want to keep going because it tastes so good, think about why you want to keep going and be honest with yourself. Food can really only fulfill one need - hunger. That is it. Food might temporarily meet needs for security, safety, comfort, and companionship, but the fulfillment won't last long. For an in-depth study of permission with mindfulness, refer to Intuitive Eating (2020) and the Intuitive Eating Workbook (2017) by Evelyn Tribole and Elyse Resch.

Food will never be able to truly feed your soul. Only you can do that by taking care of your soul and finding true peace and rest in God. As I wrap up this part, I would love for you to think about what needs you have asked food to fulfill in the past. Make a plan for meeting those needs in the future without using food. Freedom and peace with food are waiting for you. Can you see it? I can!

Prayer

Lord, thank You for expertly making my body and my dietary needs. You know what my body needs, and You have created me to discern what foods and how much food I need to thrive. Help me to enjoy it and use it for nourishment so I can accomplish Your will in my life. Help me to make the changes I need to make in the way I think about food and behave around it. Be with me as I practice peace with food, both now and as I grow in this area. Please help me to give myself grace and to give myself all the time I need to create lasting peace with food. In Jesus's name, Amen.

Invitation

If you haven't already started, use the examples of a personal menu, meal plan, grocery list, and hierarchy of food fears located on the resources list at the back of the book to help you create order and peace with food. When you feel stuck, pray. When you don't know what to eat, pray. When you want to eat more than you know you need, pray. Put your trust in the Lord, and He will bless you as you pursue peace with food.

PART III

Peace with Movement and Rest

CHAPTER 1

Peace With Movement

> It is for freedom that Christ has set us free. Stand firm,
> then, and do not let yourselves be burdened again by a
> yoke of slavery.
>
> —Galatians 5:1

Peace with movement means knowing that moving the body has many health benefits, but moving it out of obligation is harmful. It is accepting that, on some days, exercise will be prioritized, and sometimes it won't. It is understanding that there are seasons of more activity and seasons of less, and that is okay. It involves looking forward to movement because it brings you joy and feels good to move, not because you need to compensate for calories eaten. It is taking time to make movement a part of life but not feeling guilt or shame on days when it doesn't happen.

The Joys of Movement in Childhood

I remember playing red rover as a child in front of our family home. My team would stand on one side of the street and scream the song, "Red rover, red rover, send (whoever) right over!" Then whoever would run from the other side of the street and try to barrel through our linked arms. We would usually all fall down, laughing, as the person broke (or tried to break) the chain of arms.

I also remember running around our property playing hide-and-seek for hours. We would build forts in the foliage, climb trees, roll down levees, and skip rocks on the Mississippi River. There were a few homes in the neighborhood with trampolines and swimming pools in the backyard. We definitely frequented those homes in the summer months. We would go from the pool to the trampoline and back to the pool again.

Sometimes I miss those years of my life. I miss having the innocence of movement without the cultural pressure of "fitness." I ran, jumped, and played because it was fun, and I loved being with my sister and our friends.

What memories of movement do you have from before you knew anything about the words "exercise," "calories," or "fitness"? What did you love to *play* as a child? Did you have a Skip-It? I loved my Skip-It. What about a pogo stick? Or roller skates? I am so happy that roller skating is popular again! What did you love to do? What movement brought you joy as a child, teenager, or young adult? At what point was that joy replaced with obligation?

Movement Philosophy

My movement philosophy is very simple. We were created to move. Everyone delights in play as a child. We can remember how fun it was to experience the feelings of strength, wonder, and accomplishment that movement gave us. We can continue to experience joyful movement as adults. Movement is made even more joyful when we are old enough to understand its health benefits.

Properly fueling our bodies is more exciting when we know it will make our bodies feel good and our movement stronger. As our strength increases, overcoming mental and physical obstacles becomes easier. Joyful movement doesn't feel obligatory. Its main goal is not to burn calories or change the body, although both are consequences of consistent movement.

Feeling obligated to exercise is not helpful to us. How many times have you said, "I am going to exercise more this year," or "I am going to make sure I stay consistent and get stronger!"? You might follow through with these goals for a while by going to the gym, going for walks, or doing home workout videos. But, inevitably, it gets hard to stay consistent, and you give up. Does this cycle sound familiar?

What if we can find a way to look at movement differently? Instead of looking at it as obligatory, we can combine the innocence and joy of childhood movement with education on the benefits of exercise. In other words, we can take the fun we had as kids and combine it with the satisfaction that we are prioritizing our health as adults. It's the best of both worlds!

Take Your Mind Back in Time

Let's dig a little deeper into the innocence and carefree joy of childhood movement. In your journal, make a list of all of the movements you used to do as a child, preteen, or teen before obligation or diet culture crept in. Really think about it. All of the games. All of the make-believe activities. All of the sports. All of the bike riding. All of the digging in dirt or sand. All of the hopscotch, horse, and leapfrog games. Which of those activities were your favorites? Why did you enjoy those activities? What made you happy about those types of movements? Did they make you feel free and alive? Did you feel strong because you could do them better than your siblings or friends? Did you enjoy certain activities because of the people you were with while doing them? Did you love activities you got to do on your own, like swimming or playing golf? Did you love competing with others or yourself?

Try remembering what it was like to be in your body while doing those activities. For instance, do you have a memory of panting hard while running the bases during an important baseball game? Do you remember the smell of the freshly cut grass in your yard as you were climbing trees or playing hide-and-seek? These memories will help you relive the joy that came with your favorite childhood experiences of movement.

You might not have a lot of memories of movement from your childhood, or maybe you were unable to do certain activities that you wanted to do. Maybe you wanted to dance or play sports, but the cost was not an option for your family. Maybe you always wanted certain athletic abilities, but when you tried to foster athleticism, you were discouraged and never pursued it further. Maybe you were too afraid to try out for a team or experiment with certain sports or skills. In your journal, write the activities you were either unable to do or regret not doing. Why do you regret not being able to participate in those activities?

Now, take your lists of activities and cross off the ones that aren't possible or you would never want to do again. For instance, leapfrog might get marked off due to bad knees or because that simply won't end well for anyone involved. Hide-and-seek might be one that stays on the list. Kids, young and old, love to play hide-and-seek. Maybe you played sports, and you would like to play again. Many communities have adult leagues that are an absolute blast. Maybe you could start a league in your community.

Next, write down fun activities that you have discovered (or would like to try) as an adult. Remember, obligatory or boring activities are not welcome on this list. It should be comprised of all activities *you would want to do, even if they didn't burn any calories at all.* You would do these movements just for the sake of having fun. Examples might include hiking, swimming, ballroom dancing, paddleboarding, walking on the beach, or snow-shoeing.

Old Messages

Activities or exercises that you once used solely to change the look of your body have "old messages" attached to them. If any particular exercise has caused you to lose joy, the thoughts and motivations behind that movement would fit into the "old messages" category. If you were using that particular physical activity to compensate for eating, these activities need to be avoided until you are able to reframe them in your mind.

For instance, say a person used to love running when they were younger. They might have run track in high school and ran for fun with their buddies in college. But when they noticed weight gain in their mid-twenties, running became an obsession. It became something they "had" to do to regulate their weight. If they slacked off at times and happened to gain weight for whatever reason, they would use running as a way to "slim down again." When this person is ready to be at peace with movement again, running would have some old messages associated with it.

Now that person might say, "But I really did love to run, and I still might." I am sure they did, and I believe they could love to run again one day. But sometimes, there needs to be a rebuilding of the love of movement and a restoration of pure motivation before you start an "old messages" activity again. Joyful movement is not possible when your brain harbors a connection between that activity and feelings of pressure to lose weight or change the body.

If any of the activities on your adult list have "old messages" attached to them, I would advise putting a question mark next to them or crossing them off for now. These activities could certainly come back into your life later, but let's focus on healing, peace, joy, and fun around movement before making peace with "old messages" activities.

Prayer

Lord, help me to remember where in my story I began to believe movement and exercise was a means to change my body. Would you give me insight into how movement has been attached to my worth and value and what lies I have believed about it? Help me to see movement through the eyes of a child again. Let me be reacquainted with the innocence of moving my body for the sake of fun and joy. Give me wisdom about what types of movement I can begin doing in order to make peace with movement. In Jesus' name, Amen.

Invitation

Take some extra time to make your lists of movements you used to love. This is a great time to write out more of your story to allow the Holy Spirit to show you where your joy for movement and exercise and even sports or athleticism was tainted and jaded by diet culture. Maybe movement became obligatory because of body size or weight gain. Write about it. Get it out. Face it and allow the Lord to show you where truth can reign again in your thoughts and actions with movement.

CHAPTER 2

Motivation for Movement

All a person's ways seem pure to them, but motives are
weighed by the Lord.

—Proverbs 16:2

In Chapter 1 we remembered all the forms of movement and exercise
we loved to do as children and we began to reframe perspective
on movement. The goal is to get away from thinking of movement as
obligatory or as a means to change the body in some way. Ultimately,
if we can reclaim the joy of moving our bodies that would help create
peace with movement. I also want to talk about what might be going
through your mind right now. I would imagine you might be thinking,
*Um, hello. Exercise does burn calories, and it can change the body. Isn't
that kind of the point sometimes? And how do we separate them? It's not
possible.* If you are thinking this or something similar, you would be
partially correct. Let me explain.

Motivation is the underlying issue. In real estate, it's all about
"Location! Location! Location!" Well, in recovery from an unhealthy
relationship with food, exercise, or body, it is all about "Motivation!
Motivation! Motivation!" Motivation is our driving force. It is our *why*.
It is at the root of all we do. I believe in order to have true peace with
movement, your motivation needs to be rooted in freedom, grace, joy,

and caring for yourself. Let's discuss each one of these characteristics of pure motivation as it pertains to movement.

Freedom

Freedom in movement looks like running some days and walking some days because you enjoy both activities. Some days you might work out hard because that is what feels good, and other days you do something less strenuous like yin yoga or a slow swim in the pool.

Freedom in movement looks like taking time to rest when you need it or when life's circumstances don't allow for structured movement. Freedom also looks like trying new ways of moving, giving yourself grace to not be good at things at first, and counting all movement, no matter how mild, as a win.

Grace

Grace in movement looks like deviating from your plan as needed. You might have started a certain activity and then stopped when you realized you were too tired for it that day. Sometimes it looks like turning your alarm off and staying in bed.

Grace looks like giving yourself time to increase your endurance. It looks like adding three more minutes to your workout each time your body allows for it. Grace looks like taking small steps in building your strength. It is knowing that no matter how slow you go, you are going to get there. Grace looks like "it can't be this easy and this kind," when it really is.

Joy

Joy in movement looks like feeling accomplished, strong, and alive when you are done with your movement. It looks like a "good" tired at the end of the day. It's cracking a smile when you feel your muscles are a little sore the next day. It is moving your body in a way that feels good and honors your energy level.

Joy looks like chasing your kids around the house, playing softball with friends, a game of pool volleyball, or having a quiet morning of meditation and stretching before anyone else is awake. Joy in movement is watching your body get stronger as you experience consistent movement.

Caring for Yourself

Caring for yourself with movement means knowing that you feel better when you move consistently. It means appreciating your increasing physical strength, agility, and endurance. It means noticing improvement in your bloodwork, mood, and mental health. It means you can have an absolute blast with movement and recognize lasting changes at the same time.

Benefits of Movement

Even though we are trying to take the "obligation" out of movement, the benefits are there nonetheless. If we are successful in taking the pressure away, we can truly enjoy movement and the subsequent changes that come from it.

Here are some of the many benefits of consistent exercise:

- Strengthens bone and muscle structure
- Helps with cardiovascular health
- Increases agility and balance
- Helps to regulate mood
- Helps with better sleep
- Helps to manage blood sugar and insulin levels
- Helps to lower depression and anxiety
- Improves memory and brain function

- Helps to lower blood pressure
- Improves energy level
- Lowers risk of developing some cancers
- Helps to manage chronic health conditions

How Much Movement Does My Body Need?

You now have your list of things you'd love to do even if those movements didn't burn calories (because burning calories and changing our bodies is not the goal anymore). You now understand what pure motivation looks like. Now it's time to talk about making a realistic plan for movement.

The American College of Sports Medicine recommends for people to engage in 150 minutes of moderate activity each week (Physical Activity Guidelines). Please keep that recommendation in a very open hand. There will be some weeks when you will do 150 minutes or more of activity. And there will be some weeks where you won't—and that is okay.

If you hold too tightly to any standard, you are setting yourself up for failure. If you feel like 150 minutes of movement is super intimidating or may never happen for you, that is okay, too. For many of us, movement has been obligatory and lacking any joy for a long time. We have to restore our relationships with movement above all else, and that takes time.

Write today's date in the margin. Now, imagine what your life will look like one year from today. If you start today, and stay consistent with movement for an entire year, you will be stronger and able to enjoy the benefits of moving more. By "consistent," I mean moving your body intentionally three days a week (on average) most weeks.

Exercise is like so many other things in life. We want to do it, but we don't know where to start. It feels too intimidating. I am here to encourage you. Start where you are today. Make incremental, realistic increases, and in a few months' time you will see how movement positively affects your mind, body, soul, and spirit.

Prayer

Lord, thank you for my body and its ability to move and experience the pleasure of movement. Please guide me in how to change my mindset and behaviors so that I experience freedom, grace, and joy with movement. Help me to understand what my body needs and to listen to it. Help me to honor my body with healthy movement and enjoy this part of life. Thank you, Jesus, for this journey we are on. Please continue to show me your will for my life. In Jesus' name, amen.

Invitation

Now that you have your list of movements to try and guidelines on where to start, think about the best way to start, add to, or change what you are already doing. Think about what time of day might be best. Think about if you would like to join a gym, try a sports league, ask a friend to join you, or use movement as "me" time. Movement will be considered "in order" in your life when it is fun and filled with grace and joy. And one thing we know is that order brings peace.

CHAPTER 3

Peace with Rest

Come to me, all you who are weary and burdened, and
I will give you rest.

—Matthew 11:28

P eace with rest is knowing when to allow for days, weeks, or seasons with no planned exercise. When big changes happen (e.g., job changes, moving, a death in the family, births, injuries, or other physical or mental ailments), it's knowing that more physical rest might be required in the immediate future.

Peace with rest means listening to the demands of your body for physical healing and regeneration before it is able to exercise and move again in a consistent manner. It is not having guilt over giving your body the time it needs to "catch its breath" so it can continue on. It is knowing that rest begets rest, and energy and life are the results of rest.

Rest Philosophy

When it comes to rest, my philosophy was first modeled by God when He gave us Sabbath. I love the Sabbath. I love that God created the whole earth and everything in it in six days, and then He rested. God chose to rest, pause, and enjoy what He had made, even though He is

God and doesn't need rest. He paused to enjoy his handiwork, and He commands us to do the same. Every time God gives us a boundary, it is for our good. And the Sabbath—keeping one day without any work as a dedication to God—is a boundary He has set for us. It is most definitely for our good.

God made us, and He knows that we need pause, margin, and rest for our bodies and souls. He knows that we can do more with six days a week of work and one day of rest than we can do with seven days of work and no rest. If you are not taking a Sabbath day every week to relax without doing any money-making work, you are missing out on one of God's greatest blessings. Rest begets rest, but it also allows us to work harder, more efficiently, and with more joy because we are not exhausted all the time.

Whether we like it or not, we need rest. And if we don't like it, it is a sign that we aren't fully trusting God. God-made movement and rest (also called work and Sabbath) have a cyclical relationship. They are equally dependent on each other to be enjoyed to the fullest. Movement supports rest as rest supports movement. They are both needed for the absolute health of the body and soul.

Are You Getting Enough Rest?

If you feel tired all the time, please look at your work-rest habits. Evaluate how many days a week you are working, and be honest about what your body's needs are in regard to rest. Many of you, if you are honest, might say that you have not rested (*really rested*) in months or even years. If that is the case, before you incorporate consistent movement and exercise, please allow your body to rest.

You might have been very consistent with movement for many seasons in your life, but you are not resting enough. Some of you have experienced a compulsive relationship with exercise in which you feel guilty if you rest. If that is the case, you have to challenge this inappropriate guilt and allow yourself proper rest. You may even need to take a few weeks or months off from movement altogether to reset. This will send a message to your body that you are paying attention and you are willing to allow it the proper rest it needs.

The Importance of Sleep

During my initial meeting with a client, one of the first things I ask is, "How much sleep do you get each night, and is it restful or restless?" If they get less than seven or eight hours of sleep every night (nine or more for teenagers), I always circle back to it at the end of the assessment. I tell them that adequate sleep is going to be one of the first goals we will make. Sleep is essential for the body to heal, restore, and rebuild strength.

Adequate nutrition allows for the body to sleep well, and proper sleep allows for the body to utilize nutrients to nourish and heal our bodies. This is a cyclical pattern that we need each day. Ideally, we sleep well, we wake, and we eat in a consistent and honoring fashion. Then, our bodies are satisfied and able to sleep well again that night. Disruptions in sleep can cause a lot of trouble for us in the areas of food and movement. Inadequate sleep also negatively affects cognition and emotion regulation.

The majority of research about healthy sleep supports having a consistent bedtime routine. That may look like showering, cleaning your face, brushing and flossing your teeth, and climbing into bed to read a chapter before sleeping. It could also consist of stretching, meditating, praying, or many other things. If you don't have a consistent bedtime routine, try to create one. Most importantly, turn off all screens at least twenty minutes before trying to sleep. This will allow your body to relax without stimulation and give your mind peace before trying to sleep.

Ways to Rest Besides Sleeping

Sleep is not the only way to find rest. Rest includes any way you utilize relaxation to care for the body. I am referring to the times throughout your day when you are not physically active or busy. It is taking the time to pause, catch your breath, check in with your body, and ask yourself what you need. You can meet one of your body's needs at that moment or make a mental note to meet it later.

Rest can mean different things to different people. For example, reading might be restful to your spouse but might feel like work for you. You might find rest by taking a drive, listening to music, or listening to the birds outside. What do you do to recharge? Do not feel guilty taking the time to do what feels restful to you.

Many people don't get enough sleep or rest. There seems to be an obsession with the daily "grind," especially in American culture. We often run from one thing to the next and do not make a conscious effort to rest. If this is you, it is time to reevaluate and create some space for rest.

Rest is also an essential part of finding the motivation for joyful movement. If you read the chapter about movement and you said, "Yeah, nothing about that sounds even remotely fun or joyful," then you are likely in need of a season of rest. Even if you have not exercised for years, you could still be in need of the biggest, longest deep breath of your life.

When our bodies, minds, souls, and spirits do not experience consistent rest, we are constantly working from a place of fatigue and burnout. It is time to create some margin and rest. We have to make peace with rest. We have to admit where we need work in this area, put rest in its proper place in our lives, and allow ourselves to be restored. Will you do that with me? I sure hope so!

Prayer

Lord, You made me. You know how much sleep and rest I need. Lord, please help me to have better boundaries with sleep, and rest. Give me creative ideas to establish habits of rest. Please give me wisdom, Lord, about what my body needs, and help me to not get caught up in culture's reliance on work. Help me remember that my fulfillment comes from You alone, not what I can produce or accomplish in and of myself. Give me the humility to listen to my body and give it what it needs. Help me to make peace with rest. In Jesus's name, Amen.

Invitation

Pay attention to how you spend the last twenty minutes of your day before you get into bed. Allow yourself time without screens to do something relaxing and peaceful before you try to sleep. If you are willing, please be honest about how much rest you allow in your day and week. Are you taking breaks from work? Are you allowing yourself margins to enjoy, play, and do things that are life-giving? Are you always running hard from one thing to the next, or do you have a rhythm of work and rest in your life? If you would like to, write some goals in your journal for sleep and rest to allow you to create order and peace in these areas.

PART IV

Peace with Body Image

CHAPTER 1

Created In His Image

Therefore, since we are surrounded by such a great cloud of witnesses, let us throw off everything that hinders and the sin that so easily entangles. And let us run with perseverance the race marked out for us, fixing our eyes on Jesus, the pioneer and perfecter of faith. For the joy set before him he endured the cross, scorning its shame, and sat down at the right hand of the throne of God.

—Hebrews 12:1–2

Peace with body image happens when you come to a place of acceptance, and even enjoyment, of all that your body is. You appreciate its functionality and aren't bothered by whether or not it aligns with the beauty standards of the world. It is realizing that thinness or fitness does not define your worth and value. Peace with your body is simply doing your best to take proper care of your body, but not measuring your success based on pounds or inches lost. It means letting go of trying to control your body. It means treating your body with respect and appreciation rather than as the enemy.

Most people think body image is what someone actually looks like, but it's not. Body image is *how you feel about your body*. It's how the body is perceived and thought of by the one who inhabits it. If you feel uncomfortable in your own skin, it is not because there is something wrong with your body. The untruthful messages you have received about your body have shaped your body image in a negative and harmful way.

Finding Peace Can Feel Like War

There are a lot of people in this world who are heavily invested in you not being okay with your body. They are making an enormous amount of money off your disapproval of yourself.

Additionally, there are forces at work in the spiritual realm which we cannot see. These spiritual forces are at war over our innermost needs for significance, belonging, and approval. The good news is that we have the ability to fight this war and win. In the Bible, Paul states that we do not wage war as the world does:

> For though we live in the world, we do not wage war as the world does. The weapons we fight with are not the weapons of the world. On the contrary, they have divine power to demolish strongholds. We demolish arguments and every pretension that sets itself up against the knowledge of God, and we take captive every thought to make it obedient to Christ.
>
> —2 Corinthians 10:3-5

So far, we have talked about nutrition, movement, and rest. To me, nutrition is the first layer of depth when it comes to recovery of your peace. Movement and rest make up the second layer. Body image is the deepest, heart-and-soul-level, third layer. It's the innermost motivation behind our disordered view of food, movement, and rest. Body image issues usually take the most time to figure out because they tend to be the most complex.

It is impossible to fully recover from an eating disorder or disordered eating without addressing the issue of body image. It is important to state the obvious here: most people in the United States, and in many other parts of the world, have an unhealthy body image to some extent. This issue is not reserved for people with disordered relationships with food and movement. Most people would say they dislike part or all of their body to some degree.

Body Image Philosophy

We were made in the image of God. His breath is in our lungs (Genesis 2:7), and our bodies are fearfully and wonderfully made (Psalm 139:14). They are incredible vessels of our spirits and souls. We exist on this earth for a great purpose. Our bodies are not meant to assign our value or to pass judgment on ourselves. They are simply here to carry us and move us.

We do not exist to look a certain way. Rather, we are here to fulfill the purposes God intended for us in our generation. We only have one life to live, and none of us know how long that will be. We were not created to fit a cultural mold, and we need to stop wasting this precious life by being far too preoccupied with what we look like on the outside. We constantly expect our bodies to meet our deepest needs for love, value, and sufficiency. These are needs that only God can meet, and to expect our bodies to do this will only leave us empty and hopeless.

Where Does Your Value Come From?

We can have peace with body image when we surrender to the fact that cultural beauty standards do not define our value. Diet culture, the beauty industry, and images we see in the media strive to tell us something different.

When every single actor on TV is super thin with perfectly manicured hair and clothing, what does that do to our body image mentality? It conditions us to think that is what we are supposed to look like. It is the same case if everyone we follow on social media has thin, straight bodies. We think if we don't look a certain way, we must not be the hero or heroine of our own stories. And it is wrong. That is not what real life and real bodies look like.

Our bodies are incredibly fashioned creations. To say that we should look different than how God made us shows a lack of appreciation for His creation. We are functional, not ornamental. We are here to function, live, breathe, and glorify God. That is what our bodies are for. We have to reject every power of darkness trying to tell us that God made a mistake when he created us.

Body image issues are a major distraction that Satan will use to separate you from God. He wants you to think that having the perfect body is your path to fulfillment. It's time to fight those lies with God's truth!

In order to truly experience healing in this area, body image must be separated from a person's worth and value. In other words, *even if you lost your bodily health, strength, beauty, and functionality, you should still know you are loved, valuable, and important.*

In the story of creation, we are told that the breath of God is in our lungs and that we were created in the image of God. What does that even mean? It means that we are like Him in form, figure, and, most of all, value. We are not equal to God, of course, because He has no rival or equal. But when He knit us together in our mother's womb (Psalm 139:13), the blueprint He followed had similarities to His own.

You will, of course, inhabit this body in your lifetime, but your body is not the treasure. In the womb, God did not just knit your body together. He made every other part of you—your spirit, soul, and mind. Because you were made by a loving God with great purpose and intention, your value will never change. Your appearance, skin color, or physical attributes can never change your worth.

Can you let that sink in for a moment? What do you think would happen if this truth sank down into the depths of your heart, mind, and soul? What would you do differently? How would you act differently? How would you dress differently? How would you eat and exercise differently? How would you move and worship differently? How would you celebrate, dance, live, and love differently if you knew that nothing about your body influences how valuable you are? My greatest hope is that you can internalize these truths and let them begin to define you.

Childhood Wounds

One of my clients recently told me something I have heard many times before: "As a child, I thought my body was fine. I was totally okay in my skin. I didn't know there was anything wrong with me until someone in my family told me I was not okay. Until someone told me I was fat and needed to lose weight." As children, we accept the lies given to us because we are innocent, trusting, and don't know to question those in authority over us. But you are not a child anymore.

If, as a child, you were told that there was something wrong with your body size, skin color, hair, eyes, feet, freckles, etc., give it back. I don't mean to vindicate or avenge yourself. God will take care of that, don't you worry. I mean give it back spiritually. Give back every message that was given to you that something is wrong with your body. *Give it back, let it go, and take back your power.*

Another way to look at this "giving back" is to actually break agreements you have made. When we are children, we agree with lies not knowing they are lies. As adults, and with the wisdom and power of God, we can give back all of the worthless things we were given and break agreements we have made with the lies of the enemy.

Control What You Can

The only thing that you can control in this life are your actions and your reactions to what you are given. You can't control your family members, friends, coworkers, or anyone else. But your reaction to criticism is completely within your control. Unfriend people who are toxic with food, movement, rest, or body image. Unfollow their accounts. Stop the ads. Only watch shows that celebrate body diversity. Leave the friend groups. Go play with the kids at the family and holiday events instead of listening to everyone's diet plans for the New Year. Set the boundaries. Protect your heart and don't accept the toxic I-will-never-be-valuabl e-until-I-reach-an-unattainable-body message anymore. Block the false messages any way you can.

Remember, body image is at the center of most of our issues with food, movement, rest, and our bodies. We have to stop building a fortress around the inner part of our souls with dieting, excessive exercise, plastic surgery, and every other manner to change our bodies.

It is time to stop trying to earn your value and to step into *knowing* it. It is time to change the culture. That might seem like a lofty goal, but if you change yourself, your habits, your home, and your body image, things will begin to change. You have way more influence than you think you do. And if you let these truths settle deep into your spirit, people are going to begin to notice.

In his book, *Mere Christianity*, C.S. Lewis writes:

> *God made us: invented us as a man invents an engine. A car is made to run on gasoline, and it would not run properly on anything else. Now God designed the human machine to run on Himself. He Himself is the fuel our spirits were designed to burn, or the food our spirits were designed to feed on. God cannot give us happiness and peace apart from Himself, because it is not there. There is no such thing.* (Lewis, 2015)

Every effort we make to create peace apart from Him will leave us wanting. Your diet, workout schedule, or changing your body cannot satisfy your soul. You already know this deep down. Otherwise, you would have never picked up this book. Or you would have closed it long before now.

Prayer

Lord, I have been at war with this body you gave me to live in. Help me, Heavenly Father, to end the war with my body. Help me to see how I have bought into the lie that I can seek and attain happiness and fulfillment from my body. Give me wisdom to know when I am falling for this lie again and help me to set boundaries with entertainment, relationships, and myself. Help me begin to put things in order in the area of body image. Help me to see what you see when you look at me. In Jesus' name, Amen.

Invitation

Get your journal out and write about the body image messages you received as a child, teen, young adult, and even now? What were you told about your body by unkind people or even well-meaning loved ones? What false agreements have you made with diet culture, friends or relatives? It is time to recognize more of what has shaped your body image, point out the lies and break agreements with those lies. Allow the truth God speaks to you in your time of prayer and meditation to wash over you. Invite the Holy Spirit of truth into your body image.

CHAPTER 2

Body Image Spectrum

For you created my inmost being;
you knit me together in my mother's womb.
I praise you because I am fearfully and wonderfully made;
your works are wonderful,
I know that full well.

—Psalm 139:13-14

There is a spectrum of health when speaking of body image. On one end of the spectrum, there is body hatred and contempt for the body. On the other end, there is deep respect, loyalty, and kindness toward the body. Wherever you are on the spectrum right now, there is hope to reach acceptance of your body and true, lasting peace.

Because body image is complex and sometimes convoluted with issues of abuse, trauma, and great loss, this process should be slow and gentle. Take a look at the spectrum of body image below and make a mark where you perceive yourself to be today. Then make a mark where you would ultimately like to be on the spectrum.

BODY HATRED TO PEACE

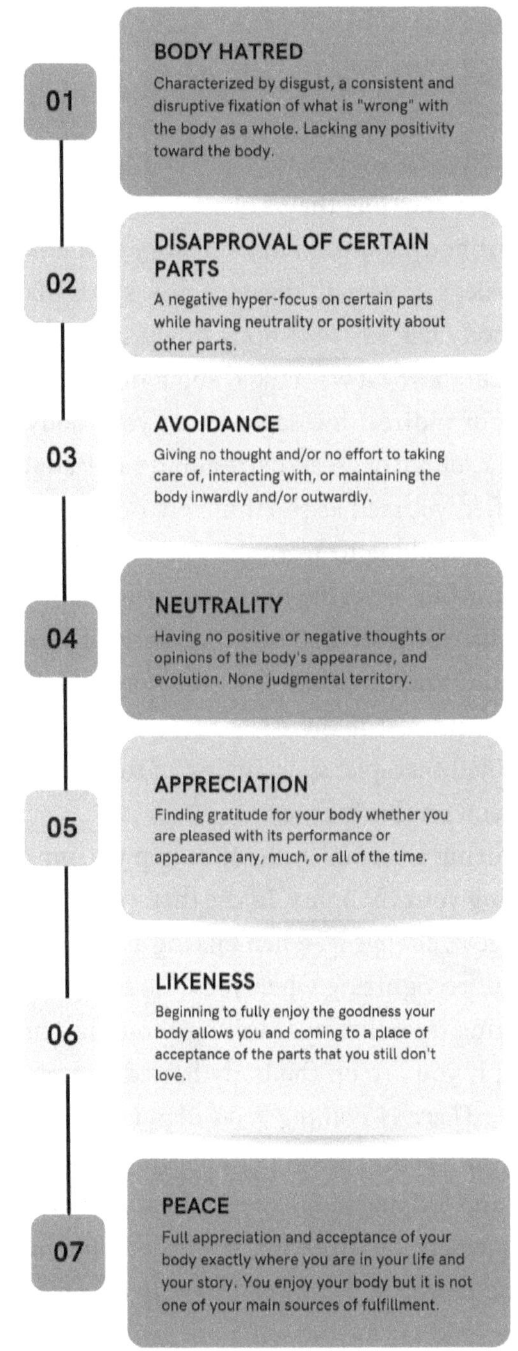

Wherever you are on the spectrum, there is hope and steps to be taken to help you move into greater appreciation and acceptance of your body. Let's look at these steps together.

Body Hatred

Body hatred is pretty self-explanatory and can come in many forms. If this is where you are starting, that is okay. It is important to recognize why you hate your body. Do you have a history of trauma? If you have experienced physical or sexual abuse of any kind, that would most certainly foster body hatred. Your body might not have been touched inappropriately, but maybe it was talked about inappropriately. Perhaps you heard direct or indirect messages about your body in some way. This, too, can be a source of great distress and can lead to body hatred.

If you identified yourself as starting here on the spectrum, please do not use this book alone to work on this issue. Hiring a therapist would be a worthwhile investment of your time, effort, and money to work on the issue of body hatred. I meant what I said earlier: it is extremely difficult, if not impossible, to fully recover your peace with food, movement, and rest if the issue of healthy body image is not recovered. A trained therapist specializing in this type of trauma will be invaluable to you on this journey.

Aside from hiring a therapist, the first step to coming out of body hatred is reframing your thoughts. In the therapy world, we like to say "catch it, challenge it, change it" when talking about changing thought patterns. It's about recognizing when your thoughts might be lying to you and challenging those lies by thinking about the truth.

For example, if you are on the body hatred end of the spectrum, you might think, *There is nothing good about my body. I hate every part of it.* First, you "catch" the thought by simply being aware of it. It means stopping and looking at it instead of letting it pass by. You then "challenge" the message by thinking, *Here is that old message again. I am hearing it and feeling it, but I don't have to take it in.* To "change" the thought, you could say to yourself, *I can believe there are some good things about my body, even if I can't name them right now. I don't believe everyone's bodies are all bad, so maybe that same truth can apply to me.* It can be a gentle reframing, but it does need to begin immediately for you to give your body image a fighting chance.

Disapproval of Certain Parts

If you marked your starting point as "disapproval of certain body parts," your first step is to investigate. Which body parts are bad? Why are they bad? What words were spoken about them by you or others? What messages have you received, and what is the source of your disapproval? What social media accounts do you follow that reinforce the idea that you need to change for some reason? And, ultimately, what need are you trying to fulfill by fantasizing about life with different thighs, breasts, stomach, arms, chin, nose, etc.? What promise and longing would be fulfilled if you worked out hard enough, ate clean enough, or paid a surgeon enough money to change this about yourself? What is at the core of your innermost soul that you need but don't have right now?

Avoidance

Maybe you are in the avoidance category. You don't hate your body. You don't love your body. You just don't pay attention to your body. Even though this is better than body hatred, avoidance can still be very detrimental. Ignoring your body is like trying to remove the heart, soul, and mind from it. It is pretending it is not there. It is denial at its finest. To hate something is terrible, but to ignore it is neglect. If you are avoiding your body, let's try to gently change this.

You can begin to interact with your body in some way, even if it is in the smallest of ways. A good place to start would be to listen to it where you previously have not. This could be with eating and movement, but also with self-care and your appearance. It could be as small as, "I am going to start washing my face more at night and applying moisturizer," or, "I haven't worn earrings in a long time, and I love earrings. I am going to wear a pair of earrings today."

Wherever you are, start with what feels reasonable, and keep putting one foot in front of the other. Ask yourself, *How can I engage with my body image or my physical appearance today? How can I stop avoiding interacting with my physical appearance today?*

Appreciation

If you are starting with appreciation, way to go! You have likely worked hard to get here, or you have had wonderful role models for positive body image in your life. Appreciation means acknowledging the good you experience because of that person, place, or thing. It is to say, "I would not have ____ if it weren't for ____." It is to have immense gratitude for something.

If you are in this place, you must think about all of the things your body does for you each day and what your body allows you to experience. You must often think about things like your strength, health, abilities, energy level, recovery from illness, etc. At least a few times a day, you consider how fortunate you are to live in the body you inhabit. You may even say out loud to your body, "Thank you so very much for all you have done for me and all you are doing for me." If you don't say nice things like this to your body, now is a great time to start. Our words are powerful. Scripture tells us that our words bring death or life (Proverbs 18:21), so speak words of life over your body and to yourself. If you are in the stage of appreciation, liking your body should not be far off.

Likeness

If you are currently at a place where you like your body (at least most of the time), way to go to you, also! Getting here probably took a lot of hard work. If you can honestly say you like your body, there was a moment in time when you decided to accept it for what it is and how it looks. There have likely been many days when you have listened to it, taken care of it, and appreciated it. Now, you have stepped into a place where you find pleasure in how it looks, how it has changed, what those changes represent, and how your body allows you to experience this beautiful life.

Peace

Lastly, if you have been able to move from liking your body to being at peace with it, then the war is over. You have stopped looking to your body to fulfill your deepest needs. You have learned to seek confidence, approval, love, and value from God rather than from your body.

You have likely been able to recognize the possible abuse, neglect, or poisonous messages linking your body to approval or value. You have been able to designate your body as a vessel that needs to be cared for so you can accomplish God's plans and purpose for your life. In essence, you have put your body image in order. And where there is order, there is always peace.

Wherever you are on the spectrum, take heart, and begin slowly working through the stages. There is time for healing. There are answers to your questions. There is peace with body image waiting for you in the innermost dwelling of your soul.

Prayer

Lord Jesus, thank You for my body. Thank You for my body, even if I don't like it right now. Lord, You made this body in Your image, and Your breath is in my lungs. I know I am fearfully and wonderfully made. Help me, Jesus. Help me see where I need to think differently about my body and act differently toward my body. Help me to see that some of the thoughts and ideas I have been given about my body's worth are not grounded in truth. Give me the courage to let go of the lies. Give me the strength to see myself as You see me. And most of all, give me the wisdom to accept that I will never be enough, but You always will be.

Invitation

If you would like to, revisit some of the thoughts or memories you wrote in your journal after reading chapter one in this part. See if any of these thoughts or memories need more attention or need to be challenged further. See if there are more thoughts and memories coming up for you, specifically associated with body image and how you view yourself.

Next, take a sheet of paper and divide it into two large columns. Draw a line right down the middle of the sheet. On the left side, write "LIE" at the top, and on the right side, write "TRUTH." Here you can list the lies you have been told by others or yourself on the left and the truth to debunk each one on the right. Scripture, of course, is an excellent resource when trying to debunk lies, but using thoughts and beliefs you already know to be true works as well. Here is an example:

Lie	Truth
No one could ever love somebody as big as me.	I am loveable and worthy of love no matter my body size.

Reminding ourselves of the truth is the only way we can get through all of this. This takes time. Don't give up. If you're thinking, *I know that I need to do this, but I have tried this before, and it doesn't work,* don't give up. The word of God is living and active, sharper than a double-edged sword. The Lord will deliver you in your time of need if you look to Him and do not give up.

PART V

Living in Light of These Truths

CHAPTER 1

Create a Culture of Peace

Create in me a pure heart, O God, and renew a steadfast spirit within me. Do not cast me from your presence or take your Holy Spirit from me. Restore to me the joy of your salvation and grant me a willing spirit, to sustain me.

—Psalm 51:10–12

Culture is the way we live. It is what we believe. It is how we move, play, eat, learn, speak, cook, love, and grow. Culture is what we experience as we dwell in our bodies, families, schools, churches, cities, states, and nations. It is dictated by what we believe and the convictions by which we choose to live. Culture is mostly established unknowingly over time and can be influenced in subtle ways. It can also be established very intentionally. Throughout history, culture has continued to change, and it always will. If we look at any sphere of influence, we can see how trends come and go and how culture can ebb and flow.

Changing Your Culture

As unique and independent individuals, it is important for all of us to have a clear sense of the culture in which we live. It is even more important that we evaluate whether there are parts of our culture that need to change. Culture begins with you. If you are going along with ideals, systems, or beliefs that don't line up with your personal values, it is time to start changing your culture.

What do I mean by this? Well, if you have been raised in a family where it is normal to pass judgment on others' bodies and obsess about weight loss and dieting, you need to make some changes to your culture.

I want to be clear: no matter how harmless comments about weight might seem, they can be extremely harmful. Talking about anyone's body in front of them or behind their back is never necessary or useful. If someone's weight really is a health concern, that should be discussed in a private manner with a healthcare professional. Too many times, weight becomes a hot topic of discussion in our families or friend groups. Unless there is real concern over someone being underweight or overweight, and you are either the person affected or someone who is in that person's direct and personal confidence, it is none of your business.

I have personally had loved ones come to me to discuss someone else's weight, weight loss, or weight gain purely with the motivation to gossip. My response has always been, "That is none of my business. That person is not my client." I have a strong belief that *unless I or you are invited into a useful and necessary conversation about your weight or anyone else's, it is never appropriate, meaningful, or life-giving to speak of someone's weight.*

Another consideration of culture is that when people speak in a way that elevates certain body types or demonizes certain types of food, it is always an indicator of their issues and their biases. It is never an indicator of your worth or your value. If you have been scarred by comments about your body from loved ones, it is time to let them go. They are not true, so don't receive them. And if you have let them stick on you in the past, remove them, give them back, and do your best never to take that on again.

Setting Healthy Boundaries

You may be thinking, *Well, I can change what I do all I want, but Aunt So-and-So is going to laugh in my face if I tell her not to talk about other people's bodies.* That may be true. I am not telling you to go start an argument with everyone in your family. You can't control anyone but yourself. But you have a lot of power. You have a lot of influence, and where you set your boundaries, people will notice. How you react to negative body messages will speak volumes and will start changing your culture. Here are a few ways you can make sure your personal boundaries with food, movement, rest, and body image are in a healthy place so you can begin to change your culture.

Thoughts

Your thoughts drastically impact how you feel and how you act. Most behaviors begin with a thought. And we know there are a few different places where thoughts can originate. Some are very obvious. Maybe someone in your life said something to you, or you read something that stands out to you. Other thoughts might creep into our brains from somewhere unknown.

Sometimes we are able to pay attention to our thoughts, and sometimes, they come and go softly without much attention from us. Both categories of thoughts are ones we need to address in order to change the culture in our lives. Whether your thoughts about food, movement, rest, and body are from direct channels or they are hidden deep down in memories from long ago, they are there. Your thoughts, much like your body, have a story to tell, and they need to be heard.

If you are not accustomed to attuning to your thoughts (AKA thinking about what you are thinking about), it's pretty simple to start. You just start listening to your subconscious banter. That is the noise in the subconscious background of every conscious activity you do. It is always there, even if you are not aware of it or listening to it. Even now, as I sit in front of my laptop and write this book, I am thinking about other things. I'm wondering how this chapter is sizing up and if this is making sense. I'm aware of the time and how much more time I have to write today, and I'm thinking about if my boys are having a good day at preschool.

There are, of course, times when we are fully and completely present with what we are doing, but most of the time, there is still room for thoughts to appear and influence us in the "background" of what we are doing. These thoughts need our attention. They can influence us and can lead to healthy or unhealthy ripple-effect thought patterns.

For instance, if you are thinking critically about your body, food choices, or lack of movement, or if you are judging others in any of these ways, those thoughts would need to be challenged, reframed, and changed. To be aware of something is to have the power to change it. So we have to think about what we are thinking about and check diet culture and toxic messages at the door. Based on the principles and truths in this book we have already discussed, I hope I have given you a baseline as to how you can change your thoughts. Here are a few more examples:

- You are asked by a coworker if you would like a doughnut from the breakroom, and you start to think, *No, I shouldn't eat that* or, *What are they going to think of me if I say yes.* Instead, you should assess whether or not you are hungry, if that sounds good and satisfying to you, or if you would like something else. Then respond accordingly. Challenge any good food/bad food thoughts that might come up, neutralize the doughnut, and remind yourself that there is no morality tied to food. Also, reject the fear of losing someone's approval based on what you eat. This will continue to deliver you from the fear of rejection by other people based on trivial things like what you choose to eat.
- You look in the mirror one day, and you just plain don't like what you see. Instead of saying things about your body that you wouldn't say to your worst enemy, change your thoughts

to something truer and more neutral. For example, *I may not love what I see today, but I can keep working on loving it. Today I will have the goal of thinking about what my body is and what it gives me instead of what it isn't.* You can also just cut right to the chase and think something like, *This isn't actually about my body because poor body image usually is about something bigger. Is there a need I have that isn't being met? And if so, am I projecting my frustration and grief about that particular thing onto my body? Maybe if I address the deeper issue, my body won't seem so bad.*

- You wake up in the morning and are too tired to do the workout you had planned. You need more rest so you can function properly that day. Instead of beating yourself up for needing rest, you allow yourself to go back to sleep knowing you will move your body in the way and timing that is most honoring to it as soon as you have the strength to do so.

When you start changing your thoughts and are more kind to yourself, you will change. And when you change, those around you will take notice. Truth is contagious to those who also crave it, so don't ever underestimate this work.

Words

There is so much power in our words. Proverbs 18:21 states, "Death and life are in the power of the tongue." That means what we say about ourselves has the ability to bring death (hopelessness, defeat, shame, and darkness) or life (hope, kindness, truth, and light). It means that our words matter, and they can change things. It means that our words can help or harm us and those we love. It means if we want to change our culture, we have to change our language.

I already drove home the idea that talking about weight is unnecessary and harmful in most cases, so I won't harp on that point here. I will, however, bring your attention back to my nutrition philosophy. *All foods fit into a healthy diet with variety, balance, and moderation.* This is what I personally and professionally live by and I hope it is one of the treasures you take from this book. It means that there are no good or bad foods, and so there is no morality associated with food.

You cannot earn any actual points with yourself or anyone else by eating "clean" or by following any diet. Any good, warm fuzzies that come to you by way of "Look how good I am because of my diet or my weight loss" is coming to you by way of a dysfunctional method of getting healthy needs met. Therefore, you have to change your language to reflect that you are no longer using your body to meet those needs.

Food is food is food is food. That is your new language about food. I am going to remind you that, as a dietitian, I know good and well that all foods are not created identically. They are different in macronutrient and micronutrient content. Put more plainly, some foods are more nutritionally beneficial to our bodies. However, that does not mean that we cannot eat foods that are less beneficial to our bodies in variety, balance, and moderation.

If you are going to have a peaceful culture in your soul about food, there has to be room for all kinds of foods to fit into your life on an equal playing field. This requires time, trust in your body, and all the things we talked about in part two. Your words have to reflect this. When you get it wrong, you need to be able to identify the judgment you are still placing on food and check yourself.

Start a trend of talking about food in a neutral way. It is enjoyed, it is eaten consistently, and it is thought of in an appropriate way for an appropriate amount of time throughout the day. Judging it, analyzing it, anguishing over it, and prioritizing it more than needed will dissipate as you change your beliefs and your words around it.

Because everyone seems to love to talk about dieting, you will be in the minority of people who look at food in a neutral way. And people will notice. They may even feel insulted if you change the subject, don't respond, or kindly say, "I don't think I would like to talk about that right now. Diet trends are not really my thing anymore." They will notice, and those in the audience watching your story unfold will be stirred, shaken, and inspired by your setting of healthy boundaries in this way. The freedom that truth brings is contagious.

Some may also be offended and "not here for this." Let them go. If friends or family members are offended by you getting healthier, then it's time to set some boundaries and look at those relationships differently. In some situations, it may be time to move on.

Behaviors

Once you have reframed your thoughts and language surrounding food, movement, rest, and body image, your behaviors will also start to reflect a culture of peace. Gone will be the days when you omit food groups, cut normal portions in half, track calories, and read diet books in your spare time. Your social media will be flooded not with workout plans and thin-bodied swimsuit ads but with posts about faith, politics, parenting, gardening, photography, and other important topics.

If you want to change culture with your behaviors around food, movement, rest, and body image, you have to stop letting all the opinions of other people dictate how you take care of your body. It means checking in with your body often. Closing your eyes, feeling cues, and allowing your body to gently lead. Your body has been with you from the beginning and has done its absolute best to care for you, so give it the respect it deserves. Let it guide you as your adopt new behaviors with food and your body.

Don't Underestimate Your Influence

Throughout this whole journey, we have been mostly focusing on you. We talked about your relationship with food, your exercise history, and your feelings toward your body. And that has been very purposeful. Changing your culture is about you, but it is also bigger than just you.

Addressing your dysfunction will bring you freedom, but it will also pave the way for others. As a mom, I know that one of the greatest gifts I can give my sons is to model the pursuit of personal healing and freedom. Whether you are a parent or not, your freedom is going to open doors for others to pursue and accomplish freedom.

This is not just about you. It has never been just about you, and that is really good news. Not just because other people will benefit from your hard work but because God made us to live in community with each other. He also made us to long for legacy. Everyone is motivated to make an impact on the world that stays long after we are gone. We will leave a mark on someone else's life in the span of our own.

Now let me state one of the most motivating facts about culture: If you heal, you will make a mark of healing and peace with food, movement, rest, and body image. And if you don't heal, you will still leave a mark, but that mark will perpetuate the pain that led you to pick up this book. I sincerely am not trying to shame you or cause you fear. It is just a fact.

If we give the next generation the worthless things that were given to us, the madness continues. But, if we have the courage to change our personal culture, we can give those around us something priceless. We can give them what we needed when we were younger. We can give them what we need now. We can change our culture. Will you join me?

Prayer

Lord, I acknowledge that I am powerless to control or change others, but I can control how I choose to act. Help me to act according to the truth about food, my body, and my true worth. I acknowledge how influential I can be as I follow You and focus on Your truth. I ask, Holy Spirit, for You to help me stop focusing on what everyone else says, does, and believes.

Help me to mind my own business and to make that business about You, Your truth, and Your purposes for my life. When I have hard days, help me remember I am building a lasting legacy of peace as I allow You to restore peace in me. Lord, help me to change the culture of my heart, my home, and my sphere of influence as much as I can. Help me let go of everyone and everything else and put them into Your able hands. In Jesus's name, Amen.

Invitation

In your journal, write down some of your thoughts, words, and behaviors that need a tune-up. Also, if you find yourself already creating more peace and bringing more truth into your thoughts, words, and behaviors, write down the victories too. This will help you become more attuned to areas that still need work and will help you to see the progress that is naturally coming as you invite the spirit of truth about food and body into your life.

CHAPTER 2

Be Known for Peace

> Do not be anxious about anything, but in every situation, by prayer and petition, with thanksgiving, present your requests to God. And the peace of God, which transcends all understanding, will guard your hearts and your minds in Christ Jesus.
>
> —Philippians 4:6–7

If you follow Jesus, you know one of His names is Prince of Peace. By his blood, we are complete, whole, and acceptable to God, despite our sins. Even with this knowledge, the church doesn't always get it right when it comes to thoughts on food, movement, rest, and body image. I hope the church can begin *to be known for peace* in those areas. I pray we can lead the world as followers of Christ in these areas as He leads through His Spirit throughout the world today. Scripture is always the authority on life, and we have looked at some Scripture throughout this book. Let's look at more.

> How lovely is your dwelling place, Lord Almighty!
>
> —Psalm 84:1

We are God's dwelling place, and He calls us lovely!

For you created my inmost being;
you knit me together in my mother's womb.
I praise you because I am fearfully and wonderfully
made;
your works are wonderful,
I know that full well.
My frame was not hidden from you
when I was made in the secret place,
when I was woven together in the depths of the earth.

—Psalm 139: 13–15

Our bodies, minds, souls, and spirits were designed so lovingly, intentionally, and specifically by God.

Lord, you alone are my portion and my cup;
you make my lot secure.
The boundary lines have fallen for me in pleasant places;
surely, I have a delightful inheritance.

—Psalm 16:5–6

As human beings in need of an Almighty God, our boundaries are good. We are not sufficient in and of ourselves. Anything we look to for fulfillment outside of our Creator will never be enough. The boundaries of how we look and how we were created may not be our favorite, but God can help us see them as "pleasant places." He can restore peace to us in these areas and we can trust His design and intention for our bodies.

Peace I leave with you; my peace I give you. I do not
give to you as the world gives. Do not let your hearts be
troubled and do not be afraid.

—John 14:27

The peace of Jesus is what we need. Not the peace of having a perfect diet, the perfect fitness plan, or the perfect body. Those don't exist, but Jesus's peace is real. This is the peace we, as the church, could be known for. This is what we could give to this world, just as Jesus did. Of all the people on this earth, we, as God's people, have the opportunity to run to Him to heal the brokenness in our lives. Only then can we be used by God to help others heal too.

Jesus is Enough

When we go to anything outside of Him in seeking true healing, validation, acceptance, and love, we are saying to Him that He is not enough and that what He did on the cross of Calvary was not the final say. It all boils down to this: do you believe that you are loved, saved, and free no matter what you eat or how you look? If you truly believe that, you can let go of dieting, weight loss expectations, Botox, plastic surgery, and any other method of trying to get your needs met through your body.

God will always provide everything we need in this life. He paid the ultimate price for us, and there is no need for us to live up to the standards of our culture. In Galatians 1:10 Paul writes, "Am I now trying to win the approval of human beings, or of God? Or am I trying to please people? If I were still trying to please people, I would not be a servant of Christ." Instead of looking like the world in the areas of food and body, we get to go to the Source who will never let us down and who has all that we need.

God made the body you are in right now. He made it for His glory. He made it in His image. He made it so that He could have a relationship with you, both in this life and for all of eternity. Anything in this world that distracts us from this truth is in opposition to God.

So, can you be known for the peace that God gives? As the church and the Body of Jesus Christ, we have a beautiful invitation to not be led by the world but to lead people to peace. As we practice peace with food, movement, rest, and our bodies, we can also show people the peace of Jesus in those areas and every other area of our lives.

Prayer

Lord, I want to be known for peace. As part of the body of Christ, I want others to look at my life and see order and peace. Not disorder and chaos. Help me to trust you. Help me to take this journey of peace with food and my body one day at a time. Help me to seek you when I feel chaotic and ask you to show me how to keep pursuing peace. In Jesus' name, Amen.

Invitation

Take time to journal and evaluate if your actions reflect Jesus as the cornerstone of your life. Do you truly believe He is enough for you? As you begin and continue to let go of using diet and your body to meet your greatest needs, how can you begin to rely more on God? Spiritual disciplines of prayer and meditation can increase your conscious awareness and contact with God. Simply confessing where you have idolized diet and body is a great first step. Then inviting Jesus into these parts of your life and asking Him to reveal His will for you will set you up for success every time. Pray this prayer on a daily basis when you feel lost or in need of grounding.

CHAPTER 3

The Bible, Food, and Your Body

Search me, God, and know my heart;
test me and know my anxious thoughts.
See if there is any offensive way in me,
and lead me in the way everlasting.

—Psalm 139:23-24

Unfortunately, some of the things that distract us from the truth about food and our bodies come from the church. There are many examples, but I will talk about a few of them here.

If you were to type "the Bible and food" into your favorite search engine, there would be millions of results for you to scroll through. Some of them would be based on Scripture, but some of them would be based on biases, diet culture, and all of the other useless propaganda we have discussed throughout this book. There are also a lot of Christians peddling diet culture as biblical truth when it is clearly not. It is their personal interpretation of dieting with a little splash of Jesus. Their motives may be pure, but they are leading people astray.

We all should be wary of false teachers of any topic, even nutrition. Any of us can go to the Bible, find a Scripture that supports what we want to do, take it out of context, and try to persuade others that we got it right. I believe many well-meaning Christians have done that, and I will avoid doing it in the text below. There are several schools of thought about how to look at food from a biblical perspective. I will spell out what I believe these Scriptures to mean, and I will trust you to study the Scriptures and see for yourself.

What Does the Bible Say to Eat?

In Genesis 7:2, before the Mosaic covenant was given to the Israelites, Noah was instructed to "take with you seven pairs of every kind of clean animal, a male and its mate, and one pair of every kind of unclean animal, a male and its mate." So even before the Lord spelled out specifically what was clean and unclean in scripture, this distinction was known and understood by those who feared Him.

Then, in Leviticus chapter 11, God spells out the Mosaic laws about what the Israelites are to eat and not eat. Verse 3 reads: "You may eat any animal that has a divided hoof and that chews the cud." Verse 9 says: "Of all the creatures living in the water of the seas and the streams, you may eat any that have fins and scales."

Some people of faith claim that we should still be following these food guidelines spelled out in Leviticus. They would point out that scripture is eternal and the Lord does not lie (Numbers 23:19) or contradict himself (Proverbs 30:5). Therefore, any believer, Jew or Gentile, must be subject to the Mosaic covenant, right?

On the other hand, most Christians are under the impression that these rules regarding clean and unclean foods are now null and void for Christians (because Jesus came in the New Testament and fulflled the law). If you keep reading into the New Testament, there are key passages in Acts chapters 10-15 that explain away both of these false assumptions above. Acts 10:9-20 states:

> About noon the following day as they were on their journey and approaching the city, Peter went up on the roof to pray. [10] He became hungry and wanted

something to eat, and while the meal was being prepared, he fell into a trance. [11] He saw heaven opened and something like a large sheet being let down to earth by its four corners. [12] It contained all kinds of four-footed animals, as well as reptiles and birds. [13] Then a voice told him, "Get up, Peter. Kill and eat." [14] "Surely not, Lord!" Peter replied. "I have never eaten anything impure or unclean." [15] The voice spoke to him a second time, "Do not call anything impure that God has made clean." [16] This happened three times, and immediately the sheet was taken back to heaven. [17] While Peter was wondering about the meaning of the vision, the men sent by Cornelius found out where Simon's house was and stopped at the gate. [18] They called out, asking if Simon who was known as Peter was staying there. [19] While Peter was still thinking about the vision, the Spirit said to him, "Simon, three men are looking for you. [20] So get up and go downstairs. Do not hesitate to go with them, for I have sent them.

As the Scripture continues, Peter travels with these men the following day to Cornelius's house in Caesarea. In Acts 10:27–28, it says, "While talking with him, Peter went inside and found a large gathering of people. [28] He said to them: 'You are well aware that it is against our law for a Jew to associate with or visit a Gentile. But God has shown me that I should not call anyone impure or unclean." Then Peter begins to tell the Gentiles gathered with Cornelius about the gospel of Jesus and the account of his life, death, and resurrection.

In Acts 10:44–48, it says,

While Peter was still speaking these words, the Holy Spirit came on all who heard the message. [45] The circumcised believers who had come with Peter were astonished that the gift of the Holy Spirit had been poured out even on Gentiles. [46] For they heard them speaking in tongues and praising God. Then Peter said, [47] 'Surely no one can stand in the way of their being baptized with water. They have received the Holy Spirit just as we have.' [48] So he ordered that they be baptized in the name of Jesus Christ. Then they asked Peter to stay with them for a few days.

This was the first account of Gentiles hearing the gospel and coming to faith! Peter was obedient to discern his vision from the Lord. The vision was not about food as many interpret it to be, but about the inclusion of the Gentiles into the Body of Christ. The vision was preparing Peter for the shocking news that Jesus came for Jews and Gentiles alike and that God shows no favoritism. In this explanation, we see that the assumption that Acts 10 cancels out the Mosaic law is not correct.

Going on further to investigate the issue of biblical food restrictions or freedoms, we have to study the following conversation between the disciples once they were seeing so many Gentiles coming to faith in Christ. Read below, from Acts 15:8–11:

God, who knows the heart, showed that he accepted them by giving the Holy Spirit to them, just as he did to us. [9] He did not discriminate between us and them, for he purified their hearts by faith. [10] Now then, why do you try to test God by putting on the necks of Gentiles a yoke that neither we nor our ancestors have been able to bear? [11] No! We believe it is through the grace of our Lord Jesus that we are saved, just as they are.

It continues in Acts 15:19–20: "It is my judgment, therefore, that we should not make it difficult for the Gentiles who are turning to God. [20] Instead we should write to them, telling them to abstain from food polluted by idols, from sexual immorality, from the meat of strangled animals and from blood."

This conversation between the church leaders in Acts 15 also leads to inclusion of the Gentiles. It highlights the "essentials" the Lord placed on the disciples' hearts to teach the Gentiles.

The Take-Away

The interpretation of all of this seems twofold. Number one: the Mosaic covenant and laws regarding food were given to the Jews to set them apart. They were given by God for their good, to keep them healthy, and to preserve the line of Abraham's descendants until Christ's return. Number two: When the church is started in the New Testament, the same dietary restrictions are available to Gentiles if they choose to keep kosher, but it is not *required*.

There is no scripture saying that the Old Testament's dietary restrictions are no longer required for Jews or messianic believers. Additionally, there is no Scripture that says the Gentiles have to abide by the same restrictions. There is an invitation to eat kosher (there is even an implication that eating kosher would be healthier), but outside of what is denoted in Acts 15:28–29, it is not sinful for a Gentile to eat pork, shrimp, or any other food that God calls unclean in the Old Testament.

The grace of God given to us in the area of food is this: eat freely except for anything strangled or offered to idols, and don't eat blood. That is the biblical stance on eating, as I understand it. Fortunately, those guidelines are intuitive and give us permission to focus on mindful eating (as discussed in part two).

The Body is a Temple

One of the most taken-out-of-context scriptures used by the dieting Christians is this one from 1 Corinthians 6:19–20: "Do you not know that your bodies are temples of the Holy Spirit, who is in you, whom you have received from God? You are not your own; you were bought at a price. Therefore, honor God with your bodies." Let's hone in on the part about honoring God with our bodies.

It is not honoring in any way to elevate our bodies above the Lordship of Jesus Christ. When we try to get our sufficiency, righteousness, fulfillment, or identities from our behaviors with food or exercise, all we are doing is practicing idolatry.

I have seen many believers use this verse to promote thinness or weight loss as a holy endeavor. Nowhere in the Bible does it talk about thinness as being holy, necessary, or even good. Nowhere. As a church, if we are going to be known for having peace with food and our bodies, we will be found actually honoring God with our bodies. Not peddling diet culture as the world does. Not using our bodies and our practices with food to attain righteousness or sufficiency in any way. We will be taking care of our bodies as we focus on what God has for us to accomplish as we live in those bodies.

So, yes, we are meant to take care of them. We are to steward what God has given us well. We need proper rest, enough water, enjoyable experiences with food, and joyful movement. We need to take care of the vessels we have been given in which to serve God.

However, if we look to these vessels to fulfill us, we have gotten it all wrong. Once again, it is a matter of motivation. Motivation to take care of our bodies is one thing. It is something entirely different to feel righteousness in any way based on our food choices, fitness level, or how closely our bodies look to what is deemed as beautiful by our culture.

So many times, I have wanted to call my local Christian radio stations and tell them, "Stop talking about dieting and weight loss! Stop demonizing food and stop allowing weight loss ads into your commercial breaks!" I have heard from many Christian clients that they feel frustrated when a pastor is talking about weight loss from the pulpit as if it's something that is righteous or holy.

I am not an anti-weight loss dietitian. Weight loss is a natural consequence for some people when they achieve peace with food, movement, rest, and body image. I am also not anti-fasting. But I am an anti-diet, Jesus-centric, our-worth-and-value-should-solely-come-from-who-we-are-in-Christ kind of dietitian and believer. Therefore, if you call yourself a believer, from a Christian worldview, you can have an even deeper motivation to do your work in these areas.

Prayer

Lord, help me be honest about my motivation toward food and movement. Give me courage, God, to admit where I have gotten it wrong. Help me to see if I have used scripture out of context to support dysfunction. Help me to use my faith to fuel my efforts for peace. See if there is any offensive way in me regarding my faith and my relationship with food and body and lead me in the way everlasting. In Jesus' name, Amen.

Invitation

This is a great time to evaluate if you have been led to dysfunctional behaviors with food, movement, rest, and body image due to faith-based influences or misinterpretation of scripture. Journal and recall memories if this applies to you. This would be another great opportunity to contrast lies you have believed about food and body with truth and scripture in context.

CHAPTER 4

What the Bible Says About Fasting

When you fast, do not look somber as the hypocrites do, for they disfigure their faces to show others they are fasting. Truly I tell you, they have received their reward in full. [17] But when you fast, put oil on your head and wash your face, [18] so that it will not be obvious to others that you are fasting, but only to your Father, who is unseen; and your Father, who sees what is done in secret, will reward you.

—Matthew 6:16-18

Is Fasting a Biblical Practice?

For our final chapter together, this is an easy one. Yes, fasting is biblical. Moses fasted, and Jesus fasted. All throughout scripture, it is mentioned as a spiritual discipline that was done by those who feared God. Any spiritual discipline mentioned in the Word is a good idea. However, we must use our God-given intellect when choosing if we should participate in certain spiritual disciplines. The Bible makes it clear that fasting is not required for salvation but is rather used to enhance our faith.

We need to be smart about fasting. If you are pregnant, suffer from a chronic illness affected by food, or have an eating disorder, fasting food would not be profitable for your faith (and would be dangerous to your health).

Ways to Fast Other Than Food Restriction

Food is what is used in the Bible when speaking of fasting. However, I believe fasting from other things can accomplish the point, which is to become closer to God. Many people choose to fast by abstaining from other things like coffee, sweets, TV, social media, etc.

I was once challenged to fast in my early twenties. I was working with eating disorder patients, so fasting food was going to be unrealistic since I ate with my patients so often. As I was telling a friend about this obstacle I had to fasting, she challenged me to fast wearing makeup instead of eating food. When I nearly had a stroke at the thought of not wearing makeup for two weeks, I knew what I needed to do. I was so convicted by my reaction and my fear of not wearing makeup that I said yes to God. It turned out to be one of the most beautiful spiritual gifts the Lord ever gave me.

It was one of the many times in my life that the Lord showed me how hard I try to meet the world's beauty standards. I was looking to culture to define my value rather than looking to God. It was a major nourishment to my soul to not wear makeup those weeks and not rely on a false sense of beauty or sufficiency. So, if fasting food is not wise for you, there are plenty of other sacrifices that would help you gain the benefits of fasting.

How to Fast From Food the Right Way

If you do choose to fast from food, follow what Jesus told us to do in Matthew 6:16–18 (see reference at the start of this chapter). This is a particularly touchy subject in the church. Many times when church staff and church members fast or talk about fasting, they end up bragging about it. It is also often used to lose weight.

If fasting food causes you to get excited about weight loss or changing your body in any way, you should not be fasting food. The point is not weight loss. The point is not to get closer to the world. The point is to get closer to God. So please, if you are someone who uses fasting for spiritual breakthroughs at times, evaluate your motives. If they are not pure, move on from fasting food, or at least wait until your motives are pure.

Prayer

Lord, I want my motives to be pure. If I fast or do any other spiritual discipline, cause my motives to be because I desire closeness and intimacy with you. If I need to refrain from fasting food for a season or forever, give me wisdom to recognize this about myself. Help me to see what spiritual disciples are purely motivated and will help me to know the truth so it can set me free. In Jesus' name, Amen.

Invitation

Have you fasted in the past with the hope and intention of weight loss? Has your motivation to fast been tainted by a desire to look a certain way? Have you seen other believers do this as well? Now is the time to repent and forgive yourself and others and to move forward. Write about fasting and ask the Lord if it is something you need to put down for now. Think about other spiritual disciples that are healthy and safe for you to do right now. Focus on those and if fasting has been used for weight loss in the past, continue to ask the Holy Spirit about it. If fasting food or other things is ever something that would benefit you spiritually, you will know it.

CONCLUSION

True and Lasting Peace in God

Wherever you were when you started reading this book, I hope you are better off now. I hope you are filled with wisdom, insight, hope, and a God-given power to heal and move forward. That is what Jesus has for us as the church and what He has for anyone who chooses to trust Him with their lives. It is not a gimmick or a cheesy everything-is-going-to-be-perfect-if-you-follow-Jesus antidote for life's problems. You will still have plenty of problems, but you will have peace in spite of them. Go to the Source that can actually help you solve them.

As we end our journey together, may we each find peace in Jesus as we walk through this life. This world, diet culture, your family, your friends, and, unfortunately, even the church, will offer you a list of temptations to go to outside of Jesus to meet your needs. I hope your soul has been fed by reading this book, and you have found evidence of God's goodness, love, power, and invitation for you to be at peace. He made you, He knows you, and in every area of your life—including with food, movement, rest, and body image—He wants you to find your peace in Him. May the Prince of Peace be with you always, and may you find in Him all you need to be at peace with your body and your soul.

ACKNOWLEDGEMENTS

This book would not have been possible without the unconditional love and support of my husband and partner, Keith. Sweetheart, thank you. Your belief in me, and your trust in God is why this book exists. I am so thankful for your support and constant companionship on this journey.

To our boys, Bennett and Anderson, you are the most beautiful part of our life and one of the main reasons I wanted to write this book. Your existence in this world gives us so much joy and meaning. May this book be a legacy of freedom to you with food and body. May you always know your significance and belonging rest fully in God's love for you.

To EJL, I would have never known one little letter would have turned into all this. Thank you for trusting me with your story and your pain. You represent what God can do with an honest and willing heart. And thank you for giving me the highest compliment, "You fed my body, but you also fed my soul."

To the Lord Jesus Christ, I have nothing without you and apart from you I can do no good thing. Thank you for calling me, using me, and equipping me to be part of your body. Thank you for filling me with your Holy Spirit and for giving me the words to write. Whatever may come of this book, all the glory belongs to you.

REFERENCES

Alfred Adler: Theory and application. (n.d.). Retrieved November 16, 2022, from https://www.alfredadler.edu/about/alfred-adler-theory-application/

American Psychiatric Association. (2022). *Diagnostic and Statistical Manual of Mental Disorders* (5th ed.).

Caffeine: How much is too much? (2022, March 19). Retrieved November 16, 2022, from https://www.mayoclinic.org/healthy-lifestyle/nutrition-and-healthy-eating/in-depth/caffeine/art-20045678

Cunnington, H. (n.d.). Instagram. Retrieved November 11, 2022, from https://www.instagram.com/havilahcunnington/?hl=en.

IFS Institute. (2019). *Dr. Richard Schwartz explains Internal Family Systems (IFS). YouTube.* Retrieved from https://www.youtube.com/watch?v=DdZZ7sTX840.

Lewis, C. S. (2015). *Mere Christianity* (Revised). HarperOne.

Physical Activity Guidelines. American College of Sports Medicine. (n.d.). Retrieved November 13, 2022, from https://www.acsm.org/education-resources/trending-topics-resources/physical-activity-guidelines#:~:text=ACSM%20and%20CDC%20recommendations%20state,on%20three%20days%20per%20week.

Richard C. Schwartz, Ph.D. - The Founder of Internal Family Systems. IFS Institute. (n.d.). Retrieved November 11, 2022, from https://ifs-institute.com/about-us/richard-c-schwartz-phd.

Thompson, C. (2021). *Soul of shame: Retelling the stories we believe about ourselves.* S.l.: Readhowyouwant.

Tribole, E., & Resch, E. (2017). *The Intuitive Eating Workbook: Ten Principles for Nourishing a Healthy Relationship with Food.* New Harbinger Publications.

Tribole, E., & Resch, E. (2020). *Intuitive Eating* (4th ed.). St. Martin's Essentials.

RESOURCE LIST

How to Find a Therapist and Dietitian

Recommended websites:

- www.psychologytoday.com
- www.healthprofs.com
- www.eddietitians.com

To access resources mentioned in Part II including, hierarchy of food fears, personal menu, weekly meal plan, and grocery list please visit:

https://www.etsy.com/shop/bodyandsoulRDapparel.